POTS SYNDROME DIET COOKBOOK FOR BEGINNERS

Simple and Nutritious Meals to Ease POTS Symptoms

Dr. Melissa R. Steven

INTRODUCTION

Welcome to the POTS Syndrome Diet Cookbook for Beginners. This book is designed to be a comprehensive guide to help you manage Postural Orthostatic Tachycardia Syndrome (POTS) through diet and nutrition. Whether you've recently been diagnosed or have been living with POTS for some time, this cookbook offers practical advice, delicious recipes, and a supportive community to help you navigate your journey to better health.

Understanding POTS Syndrome

POTS is a complex condition that affects the autonomic nervous system, leading to a variety of symptoms, including dizziness, rapid heart rate, fatigue, and digestive issues. These symptoms can make everyday activities challenging and significantly impact your quality of life. While there is no cure for POTS, managing your diet can play a crucial role in alleviating symptoms and improving your overall well-being.

The Role of Diet in Managing POTS

Dietary changes can have a profound effect on managing POTS symptoms. Proper nutrition helps maintain stable blood pressure, ensures adequate hydration, and supports overall health. By focusing on specific nutrients, avoiding common dietary triggers, and adopting a balanced eating plan, you can reduce the severity of your symptoms and enhance your energy levels.

Getting Started

This cookbook is structured to provide you with all the information you need to start a POTS-friendly diet. The chapters begin with an overview of POTS and the importance of diet in its management. You'll find practical tips for meal planning, grocery shopping, and preparing meals that are both nutritious and delicious.

Delicious Recipes for Every Meal

We've included a variety of recipes that cater to different tastes and dietary needs. From energizing breakfasts and satisfying lunches to nourishing dinners and healthy snacks, each recipe is designed to provide essential nutrients while being easy to prepare. Special attention is given to hydration, as staying well-hydrated is crucial for managing POTS.

Living Well with POTS

Beyond recipes, this book offers lifestyle tips to help you manage POTS more effectively. You'll find advice on exercise, stress management, and sleep—key components of a holistic approach to managing your condition. We also provide guidance on dining out, making it easier to maintain your diet even when you're away from home.

Staying Motivated and Connected

Managing a chronic condition like POTS can be challenging, but you don't have to do it alone. This cookbook encourages you to build a support network, stay informed through continuing education, and find motivation in the progress you make. With the right tools and support, you can lead a fulfilling life despite the challenges of POTS.

We hope this cookbook becomes a valuable resource for you. Our goal is to empower you with knowledge and practical solutions that make managing POTS through diet not only possible but enjoyable. Here's to better health and delicious meals!

Welcome to your journey towards a healthier, more balanced life with POTS. Let's get cooking!

TABLE OF CONTENTS

Chapter 1: Understanding POTS Syndrome

1.1 What is POTS Syndrome?

Postural Orthostatic Tachycardia Syndrome (POTS) is a disorder of the autonomic nervous system that predominantly affects blood flow. The autonomic nervous system controls many involuntary body functions, including heart rate, blood pressure, and digestion. POTS is characterized by an excessive increase in heart rate that occurs when moving from a lying down to a standing up position, frequently joined by a scope of different side effects that can essentially influence day to day existence.

Key Features of POTS:

- ❖ Orthostatic Intolerance: This is the hallmark of POTS, where patients experience symptoms upon standing that are relieved when they lie down. These side effects incorporate discombobulation, dazedness, and blacking out.
- ❖ Tachycardia: An abnormally rapid heart rate is a primary symptom. Upon standing, the heart rate increases significantly, often by more than 30 beats per minute (or over 120 beats per minute) within the first 10 minutes of standing.
- ❖ Other Symptoms: POTS can also cause fatigue, headaches, brain fog, chest pain, shortness of breath, and gastrointestinal issues such as nausea and bloating. These symptoms can vary widely from person to person and can be influenced by factors like dehydration, stress, and diet.

Impact on Daily Life:
Living with POTS can be challenging due to the unpredictability and variety of symptoms. It can affect one's ability to perform everyday activities, attend work or school, and maintain social relationships. However, with proper management strategies, many individuals with POTS can lead fulfilling lives.

POTS is a complex and often debilitating condition that affects the autonomic nervous system, leading to significant increases in heart rate upon standing and a variety of other symptoms. Understanding POTS is the first step towards managing it effectively, and this book aims to provide you with the knowledge and tools to do just that.

1.2 Symptoms and Diagnosis

Postural Orthostatic Tachycardia Syndrome (POTS) manifests with a wide range of symptoms, primarily related to the body's difficulty in regulating blood flow and maintaining blood pressure upon standing. These symptoms can vary greatly in severity and combination, often fluctuating throughout the day or triggered by specific activities.

Common Symptoms:

- ❖ Dizziness and Lightheadedness: A frequent complaint, especially when transitioning from sitting or lying down to standing.
- ❖ Fatigue: Chronic, debilitating fatigue that can interfere with daily activities.
- ❖ Palpitations: Familiarity with a fast or unpredictable heartbeat.
- ❖ Chest Pain: Can range from mild discomfort to severe pain, sometimes mistaken for cardiac issues.
- ❖ Shortness of Breath: Difficulty in breathing or feeling breathless upon minimal exertion.
- ❖ Brain Fog: Cognitive difficulties such as trouble concentrating, memory lapses, and mental fatigue.
- ❖ Headaches: Often described as migraines or tension-type headaches.
- ❖ Gastrointestinal Problems: Nausea, bloating, constipation, and diarrhea are common, reflecting autonomic dysfunction in the digestive tract.
- ❖ Exercise Intolerance: Reduced ability to perform physical activities, often due to rapid heart rate and fatigue.
- ❖ Cold Extremities: Hands and feet that frequently feel cold due to poor blood circulation.

Diagnosis of POTS Syndrome

Diagnosing POTS can be challenging due to its diverse and overlapping symptoms with other conditions. A comprehensive evaluation by a healthcare professional, often a cardiologist or neurologist, is crucial for an accurate diagnosis.

Diagnostic Criteria:

- ❖ Heart Rate Increase: A key diagnostic criterion is an increase in heart rate of more than 30 beats per minute within 10 minutes of standing (or over 40 beats per minute in adolescents), without a significant drop in blood pressure.
- ❖ Duration of Symptoms: Symptoms should have been present for at least 6 months.
- ❖ Absence of Other Causes: Other conditions that might cause similar symptoms, such as dehydration, hyperthyroidism, or anemia, need to be ruled out.

Diagnostic Tests:.

- ❖ Tilt Table Test: The best quality level for diagnosing POTS. The patient is strapped to a table that tilts them from a lying to a standing position while monitoring heart rate and blood pressure.
- ❖ Active Stand Test: Similar to the tilt table test, but the patient stands up from a lying position, and heart rate and blood pressure are measured over several minutes.
- ❖ Blood Tests: To rule out other conditions, blood tests may be conducted to check for anemia, thyroid function, electrolyte levels, and markers of inflammation.
- ❖ Autonomic Function Tests: These tests evaluate the autonomic nervous system's function and may include tests for sweating, heart rate variability, and blood pressure responses to various stimuli.

Other Considerations:

- ❖ Medical History: A detailed history, including symptom patterns, triggers, and family history of similar conditions, helps guide the diagnostic process.
- ❖ Physical Examination: A thorough physical exam to check for other signs of autonomic dysfunction or related conditions.

The diverse symptoms of POTS, ranging from cardiovascular to cognitive and gastrointestinal issues, make it a complex condition to diagnose. Understanding these symptoms and undergoing appropriate diagnostic tests are crucial steps towards effective management. Early and accurate diagnosis can lead to better symptom control and improved quality of life for individuals with POTS.

1.3 The Role of Diet in Managing POTS

Diet plays a critical role in managing Postural Orthostatic Tachycardia Syndrome (POTS). Proper nutrition can help stabilize blood pressure, improve hydration, and reduce the severity of symptoms. While there is no one-size-fits-all diet for POTS, certain dietary strategies have been found to be particularly beneficial for managing this condition.

1. Importance of Hydration

One of the most significant aspects of managing POTS is maintaining adequate hydration. Dehydration can exacerbate symptoms such as dizziness, lightheadedness, and tachycardia. To ensure proper hydration:

- ❖ Drink Plenty of Fluids: Aim for at least 2-3 liters of water per day. This sum might shift relying upon individual requirements and action levels.
- ❖ Electrolyte Drinks: Incorporate electrolyte-rich beverages to help maintain a proper balance of sodium, potassium, and other vital minerals. These can include sports drinks, coconut water, and homemade electrolyte solutions.

2. Increased Salt Intake

For many POTS patients, increasing salt intake can help retain fluids and raise blood volume, which can alleviate symptoms related to low blood pressure and poor circulation.

- ❖ Salt-Rich Foods: Incorporate foods naturally high in salt, such as pickles, olives, salted nuts, and pretzels.
- ❖ Salt Supplements: Some individuals may benefit from salt tablets or adding extra salt to their meals. However, it's important to do this under medical supervision to avoid potential complications like hypertension.

3. Balanced Meals

Eating balanced meals that include a mix of macronutrients (carbohydrates, proteins, and fats) can help maintain stable blood sugar levels and provide sustained energy throughout the day.

- ❖ Complex Carbohydrates: Opt for whole grains, legumes, and vegetables that provide slow-releasing energy and avoid spikes in blood sugar.
- ❖ Lean Proteins: Include sources of lean protein such as chicken, fish, tofu, and beans to support muscle function and overall health.
- ❖ Healthy Fats: Incorporate healthy fats from sources like avocados, nuts, seeds, and olive oil to promote satiety and support brain function.

4. Frequent, Small Meals

Large meals can sometimes worsen POTS symptoms by diverting blood to the digestive system and causing a drop in blood pressure. Eating smaller, more frequent meals can help manage this issue.

- ❖ Meal Timing: Aim for 5-6 small meals or snacks throughout the day rather than 2-3 large meals.
- ❖ Balanced Snacks: Keep balanced snacks on hand, such as yogurt with fruit, a handful of nuts, or a small protein bar.

5. Avoiding Dietary Triggers

Certain foods and beverages can trigger or worsen POTS symptoms. Identifying and avoiding these triggers can help in managing the condition more effectively.

- ❖ Caffeine: Caffeine can cause dehydration and increase heart rate, which may exacerbate symptoms. Limit or avoid coffee, tea, and caffeinated sodas.

- ❖ Alcohol: Alcohol can lead to dehydration and a drop in blood pressureIt's ideal to restrict or keep away from liquor utilization.
- ❖ High-Sugar Foods: Foods high in sugar can cause rapid spikes and drops in blood sugar levels, leading to increased fatigue and dizziness.

6. Gut Health

Many POTS patients experience gastrointestinal symptoms such as bloating, nausea, and constipation. Supporting gut health can help alleviate these symptoms.

- ❖ Fiber: Include plenty of fiber-rich foods such as fruits, vegetables, and whole grains to promote healthy digestion.
- ❖ Probiotics: Consuming probiotic-rich foods like yogurt, kefir, and fermented vegetables can support a healthy gut microbiome.

7. Personalized Approach

While these general dietary guidelines can benefit many POTS patients, individual responses to dietary changes can vary. It's important to work with a healthcare provider or a registered dietitian to develop a personalized nutrition plan tailored to your specific needs and symptoms.

Diet is a powerful tool in managing POTS. By focusing on hydration, balanced nutrition, and avoiding potential triggers, individuals with POTS can experience significant improvements in their symptoms and overall quality of life. This book will provide you with a variety of recipes and meal plans designed to support your health and help you navigate the complexities of living with POTS.

Chapter 2: Getting Started with a POTS-Friendly Diet

2.1 Basic Principles of a POTS Diet

Managing POTS through diet involves adopting specific dietary strategies to help mitigate symptoms and improve overall health. These principles are designed to support blood volume, stabilize blood pressure, and ensure adequate nutrient intake.

1. Emphasize Fluid Balance

A primary goal in a POTS diet is maintaining an optimal fluid balance to prevent dehydration and support blood circulation.

- Structured Hydration Routine: Establish a routine that includes drinking water consistently throughout the day, not just when you feel thirsty.
- Hydration Packs: Utilize hydration packs that include a balanced mix of electrolytes to enhance fluid retention and improve hydration efficiency.

2. Optimize Sodium Intake

Sodium plays a crucial role in increasing blood volume, which can help alleviate symptoms of orthostatic intolerance.

- Sodium-Rich Broths: Incorporate broths and soups into your diet, which can provide both hydration and necessary sodium.
- Salted Snacks: Choose healthful options like salted edamame, baked chips, or lightly salted whole grain crackers.

3. Nutrient-Dense Foods

A nutrient-dense diet ensures that you are getting all the essential vitamins and minerals necessary for bodily functions and symptom management.

- Variety of Colors: Aim for a colorful plate with a variety of fruits and vegetables, ensuring a broad spectrum of nutrients.
- Whole Foods: Focus on whole, minimally processed foods to maximize nutrient intake and reduce the consumption of additives and preservatives.

4. Maintain Steady Blood Sugar Levels

Stabilizing blood sugar levels can help manage energy levels and prevent exacerbation of symptoms.

- Low Glycemic Index Foods: Choose foods with a low glycemic index such as oats, quinoa, and most fruits and vegetables to maintain steady blood sugar levels.
- Protein with Carbohydrates: Pair carbohydrates with protein sources to slow digestion and prevent blood sugar spikes, such as apple slices with nut butter or whole grain toast with avocado and egg.

5. Address Specific Nutrient Needs

Certain nutrients may be particularly beneficial for POTS patients, and ensuring adequate intake is essential.

- Magnesium: Foods rich in magnesium, like leafy greens, nuts, and seeds, can support muscle function and nerve health.
- Potassium: Incorporate potassium-rich foods such as bananas, sweet potatoes, and spinach to help regulate blood pressure.

6. Individualized Meal Planning

Personalized meal planning helps address individual tolerances and preferences, enhancing adherence to dietary recommendations.

- Trial and Error: Experiment with different foods and meal patterns to identify what works best for your body.
- Flexible Plans: Develop flexible meal plans that can be adjusted based on daily symptom variations and energy levels.

7. Incorporate Functional Foods

Functional foods can offer additional health benefits that go beyond basic nutrition, potentially aiding in symptom management.

- Anti-Inflammatory Foods: Include foods with anti-inflammatory properties like berries, fatty fish, and turmeric to help reduce systemic inflammation.
- Probiotic Foods: Enhance gut health with probiotic-rich foods such as kimchi, sauerkraut, and kombucha.

8. Lifestyle Integration

Integrating these dietary principles into your lifestyle involves more than just food choices; it includes habits and routines that support overall health.

- Mindful Eating: Practice mindful eating by paying attention to hunger and fullness cues, eating slowly, and enjoying your meals.
- Preparation and Planning: Get ready feasts ahead of time and keep solid snacks accessible to stay away from rash eating decisions that could set off side effects.

Implementing these principles can create a solid foundation for managing POTS through diet. By focusing on hydration, optimizing sodium intake, ensuring nutrient-dense food choices, and personalizing meal plans, individuals with POTS can better manage their symptoms and improve their quality of life. This book will provide detailed recipes and meal plans to help you integrate these principles into your daily routine effectively.

2.2 Key Nutrients for POTS Patients

Proper nutrition is essential for managing Postural Orthostatic Tachycardia Syndrome (POTS). Certain nutrients can help alleviate symptoms and support overall health. Here are some key nutrients that are particularly beneficial for POTS patients:

1. Sodium

Sodium is vital for increasing blood volume and maintaining blood pressure, which can help reduce dizziness and lightheadedness upon standing.

- **Sources:** Table salt, salted nuts, pickles, olives, and broth-based soups.

2. Potassium

Potassium controls circulatory strain and supports appropriate muscle and nerve capability.

- **Sources:** Bananas, sweet potatoes, spinach, avocados, and oranges.

3. Magnesium

Magnesium plays a crucial role in muscle function, nerve health, and maintaining a regular heartbeat.

- **Sources:** Leafy greens, nuts, seeds, whole grains, and dark chocolate.

4. B Vitamins

B vitamins, particularly B12 and B6, are essential for energy production and proper nervous system function.

- **Sources:** Meat, poultry, fish, eggs, dairy products, fortified cereals, and leafy greens.

5. Vitamin D

Vitamin D is significant for bone wellbeing, safe capability, and muscle strength. It can also help reduce fatigue.

- **Sources:** Greasy fish, invigorated dairy items, egg yolks, and openness to daylight.

6. Fiber

Fiber supports healthy digestion, which can be particularly important for POTS patients who experience gastrointestinal symptoms.

- Sources: Fruits, vegetables, whole grains, legumes, and nuts.

7. Electrolytes

Electrolytes, including sodium, potassium, calcium, and magnesium, are essential for maintaining fluid balance and preventing dehydration.

- **Sources:** Electrolyte drinks, coconut water, and a balanced diet with a variety of fruits and vegetables.

8. Omega-3 Fatty Acids

Omega-3 unsaturated fats have calming properties and can uphold heart wellbeing.

- **Sources:** Greasy fish (like salmon and mackerel), flaxseeds, chia seeds, and pecans.

Incorporating these key nutrients into your diet can help manage POTS symptoms and improve overall health. This book provides a variety of recipes that are rich in these essential nutrients, making it easier to follow a POTS-friendly diet.

2.3 Common Dietary Triggers to Avoid

Managing Postural Orthostatic Tachycardia Syndrome (POTS) effectively often involves avoiding certain dietary triggers that can exacerbate symptoms. Identifying and eliminating these triggers from your diet can help improve your overall well-being.

1. Caffeine
Caffeine can cause dehydration and increase heart rate, which may worsen POTS symptoms like palpitations and dizziness.

- **Sources:** Coffee, tea, energy drinks, and some sodas.

2. Alcohol
Alcohol can lead to dehydration and a drop in blood pressure, both of which can aggravate POTS symptoms.

- **Sources:** Beer, wine, spirits, and cocktails.

3. High-Sugar Foods
Foods high in sugar can cause rapid spikes and subsequent drops in blood sugar levels, leading to increased fatigue and dizziness.

- **Sources:** Candy, pastries, sugary cereals, and sweetened beverages.

4. Artificial Sweeteners
Some individuals with POTS report increased symptoms after consuming artificial sweeteners, which may affect blood pressure and hydration status.

- **Sources:** Diet sodas, sugar-free candies, and various "sugar-free" labeled products.

5. Processed Foods
Processed foods often contain high levels of sodium, unhealthy fats, and additives that can negatively impact blood pressure and overall health.

- **Sources:** Packaged snacks, fast food, deli meats, and frozen meals.

6. Gluten and Dairy

For some POTS patients, gluten and dairy can cause digestive issues and inflammation, exacerbating gastrointestinal symptoms.

- **Sources:** Bread, pasta, pastries, milk, cheese, and yogurt.

Avoiding these common dietary triggers can help manage POTS symptoms more effectively. By being mindful of your food choices and opting for a balanced, nutrient-rich diet, you can support your overall health and well-being.

2.4 Meal Planning and Preparation Tips

Effective meal planning and preparation are essential for managing Postural Orthostatic Tachycardia Syndrome (POTS). Planning meals in advance ensures you have access to nutrient-rich foods that can help manage symptoms and maintain energy levels throughout the day.

1. Plan Balanced Meals

Creating balanced meals that include a mix of macronutrients (carbohydrates, proteins, and fats) ensures you get the necessary nutrients to support overall health and manage POTS symptoms.

- **Carbohydrates:** Opt for complex carbohydrates such as whole grains, legumes, and vegetables to provide sustained energy.
- **Proteins:** Include lean proteins like chicken, fish, tofu, and beans to support muscle function and overall health.
- **Fats:** Incorporate healthy fats from sources like avocados, nuts, seeds, and olive oil to promote satiety and brain function.

2. Prepare in Advance

Preparing meals in advance can help you avoid the stress of last-minute cooking and ensure you have healthy options readily available.

- **Batch Cooking:** Cook large quantities of staple foods like grains, proteins, and vegetables that can be mixed and matched throughout the week.
- **Portioning:** Portion out meals and snacks into individual containers for easy access and to help with portion control.

3. Keep Healthy Snacks On Hand

Having healthy snacks available can prevent blood sugar dips and help manage hunger between meals.

- **Examples:** Greek yogurt with fruit, a handful of nuts, sliced vegetables with hummus, or whole grain crackers with cheese.

4. Create a Shopping List

A well-organized shopping list helps ensure you have all the ingredients needed for your planned meals and snacks.

- **Essentials:** Include a variety of fresh fruits and vegetables, lean proteins, whole grains, and healthy fats.

Effective meal planning and preparation are key to managing POTS symptoms and maintaining a balanced diet. By planning balanced meals, preparing in advance, keeping healthy snacks on hand, creating a shopping list, and staying hydrated, you can better manage your condition and improve your overall quality of life.

Chapter 3: Energizing Breakfasts

3.1 High-Protein Smoothies

1. Berry Blast Protein Smoothie

Ingredients:

- 1 cup mixed berries (strawberries, blueberries, raspberries)
- 1 banana
- 1 cup Greek yogurt
- 1 cup unsweetened almond milk
- 1 scoop vanilla protein powder
- 1 tablespoon chia seeds
- 1 teaspoon honey (optional)

Directions:

1. Add mixed berries, banana, Greek yogurt, almond milk, protein powder, chia seeds, and honey to a blender.
2. Blend until smooth and creamy.
3. Pour into a glass and enjoy immediately.

Serving Size:

1 large smoothie

Nutrition (per serving):

Calories: 320

Protein: 30g

Carbohydrates: 45g

Fat: 6g

Fiber: 10g

Sugar: 28g

2. Green Protein Smoothie

Ingredients:

- 1 cup spinach
- 1 banana
- 1/2 avocado
- 1 cup unsweetened almond milk
- 1 scoop vanilla protein powder
- 1 tablespoon flaxseeds
- 1 teaspoon maple syrup (optional)

Directions:

1. Add spinach, banana, avocado, almond milk, protein powder, flaxseeds, and maple syrup to a blender.
2. Blend until smooth and creamy.
3. Pour into a glass and enjoy immediately.

Serving Size:

1 large smoothie

Nutrition (per serving):

Calories: 350

Protein: 25g

Carbohydrates: 40g

Fat: 15g

Fibcr: 12g

Sugar: 15g

3. Peanut Butter Banana Protein Smoothie

Ingredients:

- 1 banana
- 2 tablespoons natural peanut butter
- 1 cup Greek yogurt
- 1 cup unsweetened almond milk
- 1 scoop chocolate protein powder
- 1 tablespoon rolled oats
- 1 teaspoon honey (optional)

Directions:

1. Add banana, peanut butter, Greek yogurt, almond milk, protein powder, oats, and honey to a blender.
2. Blend until smooth and creamy.
3. Pour into a glass and enjoy immediately.

Serving Size:

1 large smoothie

Nutrition (per serving):

Calories: 400

Protein: 35g

Carbohydrates: 45g

Fat: 14g

Fiber: 6g

Sugar: 22g

4. Tropical Protein Smoothie

Ingredients:

- 1 cup frozen mango chunks
- 1/2 cup frozen pineapple chunks
- 1 banana
- 1 cup Greek yogurt
- 1 cup coconut water
- 1 scoop vanilla protein powder
- 1 tablespoon shredded coconut

Directions:

1. Add mango, pineapple, banana, Greek yogurt, coconut water, protein powder, and shredded coconut to a blender.
2. Blend until smooth and creamy.
3. Pour into a glass and enjoy immediately.

Serving Size:

1 large smoothie

Nutrition (per serving):

Calories: 350

Protein: 30g

Carbohydrates: 55g

Fat: 6g

Fiber: 7g

Sugar: 38g

5. Chocolate Berry Protein Smoothie

Ingredients:

- 1 cup mixed berries (strawberries, blueberries, raspberries)
- 1 banana
- 1 cup Greek yogurt
- 1 cup unsweetened almond milk
- 1 scoop chocolate protein powder
- 1 tablespoon chia seeds
- 1 teaspoon honey (optional)

Directions:

1. Add mixed berries, banana, Greek yogurt, almond milk, protein powder, chia seeds, and honey to a blender.
2. Blend until smooth and creamy.
3. Pour into a glass and enjoy immediately.

Serving Size:

1 large smoothie

Nutrition (per serving):

Calories: 340

Protein: 32g

Carbohydrates: 50g

Fat: 6g

Fiber: 9g

Sugar: 29g

3.2 Balanced Breakfast Bowls

1. Greek Yogurt and Berry Breakfast Bowl

Ingredients:

- 1 cup Greek yogurt
- 1/2 cup mixed berries (strawberries, blueberries, raspberries)
- 1/4 cup granola
- 1 tablespoon chia seeds
- 1 tablespoon honey (optional)
- 1 tablespoon sliced almonds

Directions:

1. Place the Greek yogurt in a bowl.
2. Top with mixed berries, granola, chia seeds, honey, and sliced almonds.
3. Serve immediately.

Serving Size:

1 bowl

Nutrition (per serving):

Calories: 350

Protein: 20g

Carbohydrates: 45g

Fat: 10g

Fiber: 7g

Sugar: 25g

2. Avocado and Egg Breakfast Bowl

Ingredients:

- 1/2 avocado, sliced
- 2 poached or fried eggs
- 1/2 cup cooked quinoa
- 1/4 cup cherry tomatoes, halved
- 1 tablespoon crumbled feta cheese
- Salt and pepper to taste
- 1 tablespoon chopped fresh herbs (optional)

Directions:

1. Place the cooked quinoa in a bowl.
2. Top with avocado slices, poached or fried eggs, cherry tomatoes, and crumbled feta cheese.
3. Season with salt, pepper, and fresh herbs if desired.
4. Serve immediately.

Serving Size:

1 bowl

Nutrition (per serving):

Calories: 400

Protein: 22g

Carbohydrates: 30g

Fat: 22g

Fiber: 9g

Sugar: 4g

3. Oatmeal and Fruit Breakfast Bowl

Ingredients:

- 1/2 cup rolled oats
- 1 cup unsweetened almond milk or water
- 1 banana, sliced
- 1/2 cup mixed berries (strawberries, blueberries, raspberries)
- 1 tablespoon flaxseeds
- 1 tablespoon peanut butter or almond butter
- 1 teaspoon honey (optional)

Directions:

1. Cook the rolled oats with almond milk or water according to package instructions.
2. Pour the cooked oats into a bowl.
3. Top with banana slices, mixed berries, flaxseeds, peanut butter, and honey.
4. Serve immediately.

Serving Size:

1 bowl

Nutrition (per serving):

Calories: 380

Protein: 12g

Carbohydrates: 60g

Fat: 12g

Fiber: 10g

Sugar: 20g

4. Sweet Potato and Black Bean Breakfast Bowl

Ingredients:

- 1 small sweet potato, peeled and diced
- 1/2 cup black beans, drained and rinsed
- 1/4 avocado, diced
- 1/4 cup salsa
- 1 tablespoon Greek yogurt or sour cream
- 1 tablespoon chopped cilantro
- Salt and pepper to taste

Directions:

1. Roast or steam the diced sweet potato until tender.
2. Place the cooked sweet potato in a bowl.
3. Top with black beans, avocado, salsa, Greek yogurt, and chopped cilantro.
4. Season with salt and pepper.
5. Serve immediately.

Serving Size:

1 bowl

Nutrition (per serving):

Calories: 350

Protein: 12g

Carbohydrates: 55g

Fat: 10g

Fiber: 14g

Sugar: 8g

5. Smoked Salmon and Avocado Breakfast Bowl

Ingredients:

- 1/2 avocado, sliced
- 2 ounces smoked salmon
- 1/2 cup cooked farro or brown rice
- 1/4 cup cucumber, sliced
- 1 tablespoon capers
- 1 tablespoon lemon juice
- 1 tablespoon chopped fresh dill
- Salt and pepper to taste

Directions:

1. Place the cooked farro or brown rice in a bowl.
2. Top with avocado slices, smoked salmon, cucumber slices, capers, lemon juice, and chopped dill.
3. Season with salt and pepper.
4. Serve immediately.

Serving Size:

1 bowl

Nutrition (per serving):

Calories: 370

Protein: 20g

Carbohydrates: 40g

Fat: 15g

Fiber: 8g

Sugar: 2g

3.3 Easy-to-Digest Pancakes and Waffles

1. Banana Oat Pancakes

Ingredients:

- 1 cup rolled oats
- 1 ripe banana
- 1 cup almond milk (or any preferred milk)
- 1 teaspoon baking powder
- 1 teaspoon vanilla extract
- 1/2 teaspoon cinnamon
- 1 tablespoon maple syrup (optional)

Directions:

1. Blend rolled oats in a blender until they form a flour-like consistency.
2. Add the banana, almond milk, baking powder, vanilla extract, cinnamon, and maple syrup to the blender. Blend until smooth.
3. Heat a non-stick skillet over medium heat and lightly grease it.
4. Pour 1/4 cup of batter onto the skillet for each pancake. Cook until bubbles form on the surface, then flip and cook until golden brown on the other side.
5. Serve immediately.

Serving Size:

Makes about 8 pancakes

Nutrition (per serving, 2 pancakes):

Calories: 200

Protein: 5g

Carbohydrates: 35g

Fat: 4g

Fiber: 4g

Sugar: 8g

2. Blueberry Almond Flour Pancakes

Ingredients:

- 1 cup almond flour
- 1/4 cup coconut flour
- 1 teaspoon baking powder
- 1/4 teaspoon salt
- 3 large eggs
- 1/4 cup almond milk (or any preferred milk)
- 1 tablespoon honey
- 1/2 cup fresh blueberries

Directions:

1. In a large bowl, whisk together the almond flour, coconut flour, baking powder, and salt.
2. In another bowl, beat the eggs and then whisk in the almond milk and honey.
3. Combine the wet ingredients with the dry ingredients and mix until smooth. Gently fold in the blueberries.
4. Heat a non-stick skillet over medium heat and lightly grease it.
5. Pour 1/4 cup of batter onto the skillet for each pancake. Cook until bubbles form on the surface, then flip and cook until golden brown on the other side.
6. Serve immediately.

Serving Size:

Makes about 6 pancakes

Nutrition (per serving, 2 pancakes):

Calories: 260

Protein: 9g

Carbohydrates: 18g

Fat: 18g

Fiber: 5g

Sugar: 8g

3. Sweet Potato Waffles

Ingredients:

- 1 cup mashed sweet potato (about 1 large sweet potato)
- 1 cup whole wheat flour
- 1 teaspoon baking powder
- 1/2 teaspoon baking soda
- 1/2 teaspoon cinnamon
- 1/4 teaspoon salt
- 2 large eggs
- 1 cup almond milk (or any preferred milk)
- 1 tablespoon coconut oil, melted
- 1 teaspoon vanilla extract

Directions:

1. Preheat your waffle iron.
2. In a large bowl, whisk together the whole wheat flour, baking powder, baking soda, cinnamon, and salt.
3. In another bowl, beat the eggs and then whisk in the almond milk, melted coconut oil, vanilla extract, and mashed sweet potato until smooth.

4. Combine the wet ingredients with the dry ingredients and mix until just combined.

5. Grease the waffle iron if needed. Pour the batter into the preheated waffle iron and cook according to the manufacturer's instructions until golden brown.

6. Serve immediately.

Serving Size:

Makes about 4 waffles

Nutrition (per serving, 1 waffle):

Calories: 220

Protein: 7g

Carbohydrates: 30g

Fat: 8g

Fiber: 5g

Sugar: 6g

4. Gluten-Free Buckwheat Pancakes

Ingredients:

- 1 cup buckwheat flour
- 1 teaspoon baking powder
- 1/4 teaspoon salt
- 1 tablespoon coconut sugar (optional)
- 1 large egg
- 1 cup almond milk (or any preferred milk)
- 1 teaspoon vanilla extract
- 1 tablespoon coconut oil, melted

Directions:

1. In a large bowl, whisk together the buckwheat flour, baking powder, salt, and coconut sugar.
2. In another bowl, beat the egg and then whisk in the almond milk, vanilla extract, and melted coconut oil.
3. Combine the wet ingredients with the dry ingredients and mix until smooth.
4. Heat a non-stick skillet over medium heat and lightly grease it.
5. Pour 1/4 cup of batter onto the skillet for each pancake. Cook until bubbles form on the surface, then flip and cook until golden brown on the other side.
6. Serve immediately.

Serving Size:
Makes about 8 pancakes

Nutrition (per serving, 2 pancakes):

Calories: 190
Protein: 6g
Carbohydrates: 30g
Fat: 5g
Fiber: 5g
Sugar: 3g

5. Protein Waffles

Ingredients:

- 1 cup oat flour (or blend rolled oats into flour)
- 1 scoop vanilla protein powder
- 1 teaspoon baking powder
- 1/2 teaspoon cinnamon

- 1/4 teaspoon salt
- 2 large eggs
- 1 cup almond milk (or any preferred milk)
- 1 tablespoon coconut oil, melted
- 1 teaspoon vanilla extract

Directions:

1. Preheat your waffle iron.
2. In a large bowl, whisk together the oat flour, protein powder, baking powder, cinnamon, and salt.
3. In another bowl, beat the eggs and then whisk in the almond milk, melted coconut oil, and vanilla extract.
4. Combine the wet ingredients with the dry ingredients and mix until smooth.
5. Grease the waffle iron if needed. Pour the batter into the preheated waffle iron and cook according to the manufacturer's instructions until golden brown.
6. Serve immediately.

Serving Size:
Makes about 4 waffles

Nutrition (per serving, 1 waffle):

Calories: 230
Protein: 15g
Carbohydrates: 25g
Fat: 8g
Fiber: 4g
Sugar: 6g

3.4 Nutrient-Dense Omelets and Scrambles

1. Spinach and Mushroom Omelet

Ingredients:

- 2 large eggs
- 1/4 cup milk (optional)
- 1/2 cup fresh spinach, chopped
- 1/4 cup mushrooms, sliced
- 1/4 cup shredded mozzarella cheese
- 1 tablespoon olive oil
- Salt and pepper to taste

Directions:

1. In a bowl, whisk the eggs and milk (if using) until well combined. Season with salt and pepper.
2. Heat olive oil in a non-stick skillet over medium heat. Add the mushrooms and cook until softened.
3. Add the spinach and cook until wilted.
4. Pour the egg mixture into the skillet and let it cook for a few minutes until the edges start to set.
5. Sprinkle cheese over one half of the omelet.
6. Fold the omelet in half and cook until the cheese is melted and the eggs are fully set.
7. Serve immediately.

Serving Size:

1 omelet

Nutrition (per serving):

Calories: 300

Protein: 20g

Carbohydrates: 4g

Fat: 23g

Fiber: 1g

Sugar: 2g

2. Veggie-Packed Scramble

Ingredients:

- 3 large eggs
- 1/4 cup bell peppers, diced
- 1/4 cup cherry tomatoes, halved
- 1/4 cup zucchini, diced
- 1/4 cup onion, diced
- 1/4 cup shredded cheddar cheese
- 1 tablespoon olive oil
- Salt and pepper to taste

Directions:

1. In a bowl, whisk the eggs until well combined. Season with salt and pepper.
2. Heat olive oil in a non-stick skillet over medium heat. Add the onions and cook until translucent.
3. Add the bell peppers, cherry tomatoes, and zucchini. Cook until the vegetables are tender.
4. Pour the eggs over the vegetables and scramble until fully cooked.
5. Sprinkle cheese over the scramble and stir until melted.
6. Serve immediately.

Serving Size:

1 scramble

Nutrition (per serving):

Calories: 350

Protein: 22g

Carbohydrates: 8g

Fat: 25g

Fiber: 2g

Sugar: 5g

3. Avocado and Tomato Omelet

Ingredients:

- 2 large eggs
- 1/4 cup milk (optional)
- 1/2 avocado, diced
- 1/4 cup cherry tomatoes, halved
- 1/4 cup feta cheese, crumbled
- 1 tablespoon olive oil
- Salt and pepper to taste

Directions:

1. In a bowl, whisk the eggs and milk (if using) until well combined. Season with salt and pepper.
2. Heat olive oil in a non-stick skillet over medium heat. Pour the egg mixture into the skillet and let it cook for a few minutes until the edges start to set.
3. Add the avocado and tomatoes over one half of the omelet.
4. Sprinkle feta cheese over the avocado and tomatoes.

5. Fold the omelet in half and cook until the eggs are fully set.

6. Serve immediately.

Serving Size:

1 omelet

Nutrition (per serving):

Calories: 320

Protein: 18g

Carbohydrates: 8g

Fat: 25g

Fiber: 4g

Sugar: 2g

4. Kale and Sausage Scramble

Ingredients:

- 3 large eggs
- 1/2 cup kale, chopped
- 1/4 cup cooked sausage, crumbled
- 1/4 cup shredded cheddar cheese
- 1 tablespoon olive oil
- Salt and pepper to taste

Directions:

1. In a bowl, whisk the eggs until well combined. Season with salt and pepper.
2. Heat olive oil in a non-stick skillet over medium heat. Add the sausage and cook until heated through.
3. Add the kale and cook until wilted.
4. Pour the eggs over the sausage and kale and scramble until fully cooked.

5. Sprinkle cheese over the scramble and stir until melted.

6. Serve immediately.

Serving Size:

1 scramble

Nutrition (per serving):

Calories: 400

Protein: 25g

Carbohydrates: 5g

Fat: 30g

Fiber: 2g

Sugar: 1g

5. Broccoli and Cheese Omelet

Ingredients:

- 2 large eggs
- 1/4 cup milk (optional)
- 1/2 cup steamed broccoli, chopped
- 1/4 cup shredded cheddar cheese
- 1 tablespoon olive oil
- Salt and pepper to taste

Directions:

1. In a bowl, whisk the eggs and milk (if using) until well combined. Season with salt and pepper.
2. Heat olive oil in a non-stick skillet over medium heat. Pour the egg mixture into the skillet and let it cook for a few minutes until the edges start to set.
3. Add the steamed broccoli over one half of the omelet.

4. Sprinkle cheese over the broccoli.

5. Fold the omelet in half and cook until the eggs are fully set and the cheese is melted.

6. Serve immediately.

Serving Size:

1 omelet

Nutrition (per serving):

Calories: 290

Protein: 20g

Carbohydrates: 6g

Fat: 21g

Fiber: 2g

Sugar: 3g

Chapter 4: Satisfying Lunches

4.1 Hearty Salads with Electrolyte-Rich Ingredients

1. Kale and Quinoa Salad with Citrus Dressing

Ingredients:

- 2 cups kale, chopped
- 1 cup cooked quinoa
- 1/2 cup orange segments
- 1/4 cup pomegranate seeds
- 1/4 cup crumbled feta cheese
- 1/4 cup sunflower seeds
- 1/4 cup red onion, thinly sliced

Citrus Dressing:

- 1/4 cup orange juice
- 2 tablespoons olive oil
- 1 tablespoon apple cider vinegar
- 1 teaspoon honey
- Salt and pepper to taste

Directions:

1. In a large bowl, combine kale, cooked quinoa, orange segments, pomegranate seeds, feta cheese, sunflower seeds, and red onion.
2. In a small bowl, whisk together the orange juice, olive oil, apple cider vinegar, honey, salt, and pepper.
3. Pour the dressing over the salad and toss to combine.
4. Serve immediately.

Serving Size:

4 servings

Nutrition (per serving):

Calories: 250

Protein: 8g

Carbohydrates: 30g

Fat: 12g

Fiber: 6g

Sugar: 10g

2. Spinach and Avocado Salad with Lemon Vinaigrette

Ingredients:

- 4 cups baby spinach
- 1 avocado, sliced
- 1/4 cup red bell pepper, diced
- 1/4 cup cherry tomatoes, halved
- 1/4 cup cucumber, sliced
- 2 tablespoons pumpkin seeds
- 2 tablespoons crumbled goat cheese

Lemon Vinaigrette:

- 1/4 cup lemon juice
- 2 tablespoons olive oil
- 1 teaspoon Dijon mustard
- 1 teaspoon maple syrup
- Salt and pepper to taste

Directions:

1. In a large bowl, combine baby spinach, avocado, red bell pepper, cherry tomatoes, cucumber, pumpkin seeds, and goat cheese.
2. In a small bowl, whisk together the lemon juice, olive oil, Dijon mustard, maple syrup, salt, and pepper.
3. Pour the dressing over the salad and toss to combine.
4. Serve immediately.

Serving Size:

4 servings

Nutrition (per serving):

Calories: 220

Protein: 5g

Carbohydrates: 12g

Fat: 18g

Fiber: 7g

Sugar: 4g

3. Watermelon and Cucumber Salad with Feta

Ingredients:

- 4 cups watermelon, cubed
- 2 cups cucumber, sliced
- 1/4 cup red onion, thinly sliced
- 1/4 cup fresh mint leaves, chopped
- 1/4 cup crumbled feta cheese

Dressing:

- 2 tablespoons lime juice
- 2 tablespoons olive oil
- 1 teaspoon honey
- Salt and pepper to taste

Directions:

1. In a large bowl, combine watermelon, cucumber, red onion, mint leaves, and feta cheese.
2. In a small bowl, whisk together the lime juice, olive oil, honey, salt, and pepper.
3. Pour the dressing over the salad and toss to combine.
4. Serve immediately.

Serving Size:

4 servings

Nutrition (per serving):

Calories: 150

Protein: 4g

Carbohydrates: 20g

Fat: 7g

Fiber: 2g

Sugar: 15g

4. Tomato and Mozzarella Salad with Basil

Ingredients:

- 4 cups cherry tomatoes, halved
- 1 cup fresh mozzarella balls (bocconcini), halved

- 1/4 cup fresh basil leaves, chopped
- 1/4 cup red onion, thinly sliced

Balsamic Dressing:

- 2 tablespoons balsamic vinegar
- 2 tablespoons olive oil
- 1 teaspoon honey
- Salt and pepper to taste

Directions:

1. In a large bowl, combine cherry tomatoes, mozzarella balls, basil leaves, and red onion.
2. In a small bowl, whisk together the balsamic vinegar, olive oil, honey, salt, and pepper.
3. Pour the dressing over the salad and toss to combine.
4. Serve immediately.
5. Serving Size:

4 servings

Nutrition (per serving):

Calories: 200

Protein: 9g

Carbohydrates: 10g

Fat: 15g

Fiber: 2g

Sugar: 6g

5. Chickpea and Avocado Salad with Tahini Dressing

Ingredients:

- 2 cups cooked chickpeas (or canned, drained and rinsed)
- 1 avocado, diced
- 1/2 cup cherry tomatoes, halved
- 1/4 cup red bell pepper, diced
- 1/4 cup cucumber, sliced
- 2 tablespoons chopped fresh parsley

Tahini Dressing:

- 2 tablespoons tahini
- 2 tablespoons lemon juice
- 1 tablespoon olive oil
- 1 teaspoon maple syrup
- 1-2 tablespoons water (to thin, as needed)
- Salt and pepper to taste

Directions:

1. In a large bowl, combine chickpeas, avocado, cherry tomatoes, red bell pepper, cucumber, and parsley.
2. In a small bowl, whisk together the tahini, lemon juice, olive oil, maple syrup, water, salt, and pepper until smooth.
3. Pour the dressing over the salad and toss to combine.
4. Serve immediately.

Serving Size:

4 servings

Nutrition (per serving):

Calories: 250

Protein: 7g

Carbohydrates: 22g

Fat: 16g

Fiber: 8g

Sugar: 5g

4.2 Light and Easy Sandwiches

1. Turkey and Avocado Sandwich

Ingredients:

- 2 slices whole grain bread
- 4 slices turkey breast
- 1/2 avocado, sliced
- 1/4 cup baby spinach
- 1 tablespoon Dijon mustard
- Salt and pepper to taste

Directions:

- Toast the slices of whole grain bread if desired.
- Spread Dijon mustard on one side of each slice of bread.
- Layer turkey breast, avocado slices, and baby spinach on one slice of bread.
- Season with salt and pepper to taste.
- Top with the second slice of bread, mustard side down.
- Cut in half and serve immediately.

Serving Size:

1 sandwich

Nutrition (per serving):

Calories: 320

Protein: 20g

Carbohydrates: 35g

Fat: 12g

Fiber: 8g

Sugar: 4g

2. Mediterranean Veggie Sandwich

Ingredients:

- 2 slices whole grain bread
- 1/4 cup hummus
- 1/4 cup cucumber, sliced
- 1/4 cup red bell pepper, sliced
- 1/4 cup cherry tomatoes, halved
- 1/4 cup crumbled feta cheese
- 1 tablespoon fresh basil, chopped

Directions:

1. Toast the slices of whole grain bread if desired.
2. Spread hummus on one side of each slice of bread.
3. Layer cucumber, red bell pepper, cherry tomatoes, feta cheese, and basil on one slice of bread.
4. Top with the second slice of bread, hummus side down.
5. Cut in half and serve immediately.

Serving Size:

1 sandwich

Nutrition (per serving):

Calories: 350

Protein: 12g

Carbohydrates: 42g

Fat: 15g

Fiber: 9g

Sugar: 7g

3. Chicken Salad Sandwich

Ingredients:

- 2 slices whole grain bread
- 1/2 cup cooked chicken breast, shredded
- 2 tablespoons Greek yogurt
- 1 tablespoon Dijon mustard
- 1/4 cup celery, diced
- 1/4 cup red grapes, halved
- 1 tablespoon fresh parsley, chopped
- Salt and pepper to taste

Directions:

1. In a bowl, combine shredded chicken, Greek yogurt, Dijon mustard, celery, red grapes, parsley, salt, and pepper. Mix well.
2. Spread the chicken salad mixture on one slice of whole grain bread.
3. Top with the second slice of bread.
4. Cut in half and serve immediately.

Serving Size:

1 sandwich

Nutrition (per serving):

Calories: 300

Protein: 25g

Carbohydrates: 35g

Fat: 7g

Fiber: 6g

Sugar: 8g

4. Tuna and Avocado Sandwich

Ingredients:

- 2 slices whole grain bread
- 1 can tuna in water, drained
- 1/2 avocado, mashed
- 1 tablespoon Greek yogurt
- 1 tablespoon lemon juice
- 1/4 cup cucumber, sliced
- Salt and pepper to taste

Directions:

1. In a bowl, combine the drained tuna, mashed avocado, Greek yogurt, lemon juice, salt, and pepper. Mix well.
2. Spread the tuna and avocado mixture on one slice of whole grain bread.
3. Layer cucumber slices on top.
4. Top with the second slice of bread.
5. Cut in half and serve immediately.

Serving Size:

1 sandwich

Nutrition (per serving):

Calories: 350
Protein: 30g
Carbohydrates: 35g
Fat: 12g
Fiber: 8g
Sugar: 4g

5. Caprese Sandwich

Ingredients:

- 2 slices whole grain bread
- 1/4 cup fresh mozzarella, sliced
- 1/4 cup cherry tomatoes, halved
- 1/4 cup fresh basil leaves
- 1 tablespoon balsamic glaze
- 1 tablespoon olive oil
- Salt and pepper to taste

Directions:

1. Toast the slices of whole grain bread if desired.
2. Layer fresh mozzarella, cherry tomatoes, and basil leaves on one slice of bread.
3. Drizzle with balsamic glaze and olive oil. Season with salt and pepper.
4. Top with the second slice of bread.
5. Cut in half and serve immediately.

Serving Size:

1 sandwich

Nutrition (per serving):

Calories: 320

Protein: 15g

Carbohydrates: 35g

Fat: 14g

Fiber: 6g

Sugar: 6g

4.3 Protein-Packed Wraps and Roll-Ups

1. Grilled Chicken and Veggie Wrap

Ingredients:

- 1 large whole grain tortilla
- 4 oz grilled chicken breast, sliced
- 1/4 cup hummus
- 1/4 cup shredded carrots
- 1/4 cup cucumber, sliced
- 1/4 cup bell peppers, sliced
- 1/4 cup baby spinach
- 1 tablespoon olive oil
- Salt and pepper to taste

Directions:

1. Spread hummus evenly over the whole grain tortilla.
2. Layer the grilled chicken, shredded carrots, cucumber, bell peppers, and baby spinach on the tortilla.
3. Drizzle with olive oil and season with salt and pepper.
4. Roll up the tortilla tightly, tucking in the sides as you go.
5. Cut in half and serve immediately.

Serving Size:

1 wrap

Nutrition (per serving):

Calories: 350

Protein: 28g

Carbohydrates: 32g

Fat: 12g

Fiber: 8g

Sugar: 4g

2. Turkey and Avocado Roll-Up

Ingredients:

- 1 large whole grain tortilla
- 4 slices turkey breast
- 1/2 avocado, sliced
- 1/4 cup shredded lettuce
- 1/4 cup tomato, diced
- 1 tablespoon Greek yogurt
- 1 tablespoon Dijon mustard
- Salt and pepper to taste

Directions:

1. Spread Greek yogurt and Dijon mustard evenly over the whole grain tortilla.
2. Layer turkey breast, avocado slices, shredded lettuce, and diced tomato on the tortilla.
3. Season with salt and pepper.
4. Roll up the tortilla tightly, tucking in the sides as you go.
5. Cut in half and serve immediately.

Serving Size:

1 roll-up

Nutrition (per serving):

Calories: 320

Protein: 25g

Carbohydrates: 30g

Fat: 12g

Fiber: 7g

Sugar: 4g

3. Tuna and Spinach Wrap

Ingredients:

- 1 large whole grain tortilla
- 1 can tuna in water, drained
- 1/4 cup Greek yogurt
- 1 tablespoon lemon juice
- 1/4 cup baby spinach
- 1/4 cup shredded carrots
- 1/4 cup cucumber, sliced
- Salt and pepper to taste

Directions:

1. In a bowl, mix together the drained tuna, Greek yogurt, lemon juice, salt, and pepper.
2. Spread the tuna mixture evenly over the whole grain tortilla.
3. Layer baby spinach, shredded carrots, and cucumber slices on the tortilla.
4. Roll up the tortilla tightly, tucking in the sides as you go.
5. Cut in half and serve immediately.

Serving Size:

1 wrap

Nutrition (per serving):

Calories: 330

Protein: 30g

Carbohydrates: 28g

Fat: 10g

Fiber: 7g

Sugar: 4g

4. Black Bean and Quinoa Wrap

Ingredients:

- 1 large whole grain tortilla
- 1/2 cup cooked quinoa
- 1/2 cup black beans, drained and rinsed
- 1/4 cup corn kernels
- 1/4 cup bell peppers, diced
- 1/4 cup avocado, diced
- 1 tablespoon salsa
- 1 tablespoon Greek yogurt
- Salt and pepper to taste

Directions:

1. In a bowl, mix together cooked quinoa, black beans, corn kernels, bell peppers, avocado, salsa, Greek yogurt, salt, and pepper.
2. Spread the mixture evenly over the whole grain tortilla.
3. Roll up the tortilla tightly, tucking in the sides as you go.
4. Cut in half and serve immediately.

Serving Size:

1 wrap

Nutrition (per serving):

Calories: 340

Protein: 15g

Carbohydrates: 50g

Fat: 10g

Fiber: 12g

Sugar: 6g

5. Egg and Veggie Breakfast Wrap

Ingredients:

- 1 large whole grain tortilla
- 2 large eggs, scrambled
- 1/4 cup bell peppers, diced
- 1/4 cup spinach
- 1/4 cup mushrooms, sliced
- 1 tablespoon shredded cheddar cheese
- 1 tablespoon olive oil
- Salt and pepper to taste

Directions:

1. In a non-stick skillet, heat olive oil over medium heat. Add bell peppers, spinach, and mushrooms. Cook until vegetables are tender.
2. Add scrambled eggs to the skillet and cook until fully cooked. Season with salt and pepper.
3. Lay the whole grain tortilla flat and spoon the egg and veggie mixture onto the center.
4. Sprinkle shredded cheddar cheese on top.
5. Roll up the tortilla tightly, tucking in the sides as you go.

6. Cut in half and serve immediately.

Serving Size:

1 wrap

Nutrition (per serving):

Calories: 320

Protein: 20g

Carbohydrates: 30g

Fat: 15g

Fiber: 6g

Sugar: 4g

4.4 Warm and Comforting Soups

1. Chicken and Vegetable Soup

Ingredients:

- 2 tablespoons olive oil
- 1 onion, chopped
- 2 cloves garlic, minced
- 2 carrots, chopped
- 2 celery stalks, chopped
- 1 zucchini, chopped
- 1 cup green beans, chopped
- 1 cup corn kernels
- 6 cups chicken broth
- 2 cups cooked chicken breast, shredded
- 1 teaspoon dried thyme
- 1 teaspoon dried oregano
- Salt and pepper to taste

Directions:

1. Heat olive oil in a large pot over medium heat. Add onion and garlic, and sauté until softened.
2. Add carrots, celery, zucchini, green beans, and corn. Cook for 5-7 minutes until vegetables are slightly tender.
3. Pour in chicken broth and bring to a boil.
4. Reduce heat and add shredded chicken, thyme, oregano, salt, and pepper.
5. Simmer for 20 minutes until vegetables are fully cooked and flavors are blended.
6. Serve hot.

Serving Size:

6 servings

Nutrition (per serving):

Calories: 220

Protein: 18g

Carbohydrates: 15g

Fat: 8g

Fiber: 4g

Sugar: 5g

2. Lentil and Spinach Soup

Ingredients:

- 2 tablespoons olive oil
- 1 onion, chopped
- 2 cloves garlic, minced
- 2 carrots, chopped
- 2 celery stalks, chopped
- 1 cup dried lentils, rinsed
- 6 cups vegetable broth
- 1 can diced tomatoes (14.5 oz)
- 1 teaspoon ground cumin
- 1 teaspoon ground coriander
- 1/2 teaspoon turmeric
- 4 cups baby spinach
- Salt and pepper to taste

Directions:

1. Heat olive oil in a large pot over medium heat. Add onion and garlic, and sauté until softened.

2. Add carrots and celery. Cook for 5 minutes until vegetables are slightly tender.

3. Stir in lentils, vegetable broth, diced tomatoes, cumin, coriander, turmeric, salt, and pepper.

4. Bring to a boil, then reduce heat and simmer for 30 minutes until lentils are tender.

5. Stir in baby spinach and cook until wilted, about 5 minutes.

6. Serve hot.

Serving Size:

6 servings

Nutrition (per serving):

Calories: 200

Protein: 10g

Carbohydrates: 30g

Fat: 6g

Fiber: 8g

Sugar: 6g

3. Tomato Basil Soup

Ingredients:

- 2 tablespoons olive oil
- 1 onion, chopped
- 2 cloves garlic, minced
- 4 cups fresh tomatoes, chopped
- 4 cups vegetable broth
- 1/4 cup fresh basil, chopped
- 1 teaspoon dried oregano
- 1/2 cup coconut milk

- Salt and pepper to taste

Directions:

1. Heat olive oil in a large pot over medium heat. Add onion and garlic, and sauté until softened.
2. Add chopped tomatoes and cook for 10 minutes until tomatoes are broken down.
3. Pour in vegetable broth, basil, oregano, salt, and pepper. Bring to a boil.
4. Reduce heat and simmer for 20 minutes.
5. Use an immersion blender to puree the soup until smooth.
6. Stir in coconut milk and heat through.
7. Serve hot.

Serving Size:

6 servings

Nutrition (per serving):

Calories: 150

Protein: 3g

Carbohydrates: 18g

Fat: 8g

Fiber: 4g

Sugar: 12g

4. Sweet Potato and Black Bean Soup

Ingredients:

- 2 tablespoons olive oil
- 1 onion, choppcd
- 2 cloves garlic, minced

- 2 sweet potatoes, peeled and cubed
- 1 red bell pepper, chopped
- 1 can black beans (15 oz), drained and rinsed
- 6 cups vegetable broth
- 1 teaspoon ground cumin
- 1 teaspoon chili powder
- 1/2 teaspoon smoked paprika
- Salt and pepper to taste

Directions:

1. Heat olive oil in a large pot over medium heat. Add onion and garlic, and sauté until softened.
2. Add sweet potatoes and red bell pepper. Cook for 5 minutes until vegetables are slightly tender.
3. Stir in black beans, vegetable broth, cumin, chili powder, smoked paprika, salt, and pepper.
4. Bring to a boil, then reduce heat and simmer for 25-30 minutes until sweet potatoes are tender.
5. Use an immersion blender to partially puree the soup, leaving some chunks for texture.
6. Serve hot.

Serving Size:

6 servings

Nutrition (per serving):

Calories: 250

Protein: 8g

Carbohydrates: 40g

Fat: 7g

Fiber: 10g

Sugar: 8g

5. Broccoli and Cheddar Soup

Ingredients:

- 2 tablespoons butter
- 1 onion, chopped
- 2 cloves garlic, minced
- 4 cups broccoli florets
- 4 cups vegetable broth
- 1 cup shredded carrots
- 1 cup milk
- 2 cups shredded cheddar cheese
- Salt and pepper to taste

Directions:

1. Heat butter in a large pot over medium heat. Add onion and garlic, and sauté until softened.
2. Add broccoli florets and vegetable broth. Bring to a boil.
3. Reduce heat and simmer for 15 minutes until broccoli is tender.
4. Use an immersion blender to partially puree the soup, leaving some chunks for texture.
5. Stir in shredded carrots and milk. Heat through.
6. Gradually add cheddar cheese, stirring until melted and smooth.
7. Season with salt and pepper.
8. Serve hot.

Serving Size:

6 servings

Nutrition (per serving):

Calories: 300
Protein: 15g
Carbohydrates: 20g
Fat: 18g
Fiber: 4g
Sugar: 6g

Chapter 5: Quick and Healthy Snacks

5.1 Electrolyte Boosting Snacks

1. Coconut Water and Chia Seed Pudding

Ingredients:

- 1 cup coconut water
- 1/4 cup chia seeds
- 1 tablespoon honey (optional)
- 1/2 teaspoon vanilla extract
- Fresh fruit for topping (optional)

Directions:

1. In a bowl, combine coconut water, chia seeds, honey (if using), and vanilla extract. Mix well.
2. Cover and refrigerate for at least 4 hours or overnight, until the mixture has thickened to a pudding-like consistency.
3. Serve chilled, topped with fresh fruit if desired.

Serving Size:

2 servings

Nutrition (per serving):

Calories: 120

Protein: 3g

Carbohydrates: 18g

Fat: 5g

Fiber: 7g

Sugar: 7g

2. Watermelon and Feta Salad

Ingredients:

- 2 cups watermelon, cubed
- 1/4 cup feta cheese, crumbled
- 1 tablespoon fresh mint, chopped
- 1 tablespoon lime juice
- Pinch of salt

Directions:

1. In a bowl, combine watermelon cubes, feta cheese, and chopped mint.
2. Drizzle with lime juice and sprinkle with a pinch of salt.
3. Toss gently to combine.
4. Serve chilled.

Serving Size:

2 servings

Nutrition (per serving):

Calories: 110

Protein: 3g

Carbohydrates: 15g

Fat: 5g

Fiber: 1g

Sugar: 12g

3. Banana and Almond Butter Bites

Ingredients:

- 2 bananas, sliced into rounds

- 2 tablespoons almond butter
- 1 tablespoon honey (optional)
- 1 tablespoon chia seeds

Directions:

1. Spread a small amount of almond butter on each banana slice.
2. Drizzle with honey if using.
3. Sprinkle with chia seeds.
4. Serve immediately or refrigerate for a chilled snack.
5. Serving Size:

2 servings

Nutrition (per serving):

Calories: 210
Protein: 4g
Carbohydrates: 35g
Fat: 8g
Fiber: 5g
Sugar: 20g

4. Cucumber and Greek Yogurt Dip

Ingredients:

- 1 cup Greek yogurt
- 1/2 cucumber, finely diced
- 1 tablespoon fresh dill, chopped
- 1 tablespoon lemon juice
- 1/2 teaspoon garlic powder
- Salt and pepper to taste

Directions:

1. In a bowl, combine Greek yogurt, diced cucumber, fresh dill, lemon juice, garlic powder, salt, and pepper. Mix well.
2. Serve with vegetable sticks or whole grain crackers.

Serving Size:

4 servings

Nutrition (per serving):

Calories: 60
Protein: 5g
Carbohydrates: 5g
Fat: 2g
Fiber: 0.5g
Sugar: 3g

5. Roasted Chickpeas

Ingredients:

- 1 can chickpeas (15 oz), drained and rinsed
- 1 tablespoon olive oil
- 1 teaspoon smoked paprika
- 1/2 teaspoon garlic powder
- 1/2 teaspoon sea salt

Directions:

1. Preheat oven to 400°F (200°C).
2. Pat the chickpeas dry with a paper towel.

3. In a bowl, toss chickpeas with olive oil, smoked paprika, garlic powder, and sea salt.

4. Spread the chickpeas in a single layer on a baking sheet.

5. Roast for 25-30 minutes, or until crispy, shaking the pan halfway through.

6. Let cool slightly before serving.

Serving Size:

4 servings

Nutrition (per serving):

Calories: 120

Protein: 5g

Carbohydrates: 18g

Fat: 4g

Fiber: 5g

Sugar: 1g

5.2 High-Fiber Snack Bars

1. Oatmeal Raisin Snack Bars

Ingredients:

- 2 cups rolled oats
- 1 cup almond flour
- 1/2 cup raisins
- 1/2 cup chopped walnuts
- 1/2 cup honey or maple syrup
- 1/2 cup unsweetened applesauce
- 1 teaspoon cinnamon
- 1/2 teaspoon salt
- 1 teaspoon vanilla extract

Directions:

1. Preheat the oven to 350°F (175°C). Line an 8x8-inch baking dish with parchment paper.
2. In a large bowl, combine oats, almond flour, raisins, chopped walnuts, cinnamon, and salt.
3. In a separate bowl, mix together honey or maple syrup, applesauce, and vanilla extract.
4. Pour the wet ingredients into the dry ingredients and mix until well combined.
5. Press the mixture into the prepared baking dish.
6. Bake for 25-30 minutes, or until golden brown.
7. Let cool completely before cutting into bars.

Serving Size:

12 bars

Nutrition (per serving):

Calories: 180
Protein: 4g
Carbohydrates: 28g
Fat: 7g
Fiber: 4g
Sugar: 13g

2. Chocolate Chip Pumpkin Seed Bars

Ingredients:

- 1 1/2 cups rolled oats
- 1/2 cup pumpkin seeds
- 1/2 cup dark chocolate chips
- 1/2 cup almond butter
- 1/3 cup honey or maple syrup
- 1 teaspoon vanilla extract
- 1/4 teaspoon salt

Directions:

1. Preheat the oven to 350°F (175°C). Line an 8x8-inch baking dish with parchment paper.
2. In a large bowl, combine oats, pumpkin seeds, and dark chocolate chips.
3. In a separate bowl, mix together almond butter, honey or maple syrup, vanilla extract, and salt.
4. Pour the wet ingredients into the dry ingredients and mix until well combined.
5. Press the mixture into the prepared baking dish.
6. Bakc for 20-25 minutes, or until set.
7. Let cool completely before cutting into bars.

Serving Size:
12 bars

Nutrition (per serving):

Calories: 190
Protein: 5g
Carbohydrates: 23g
Fat: 10g
Fiber: 4g
Sugar: 12g

3. Cranberry Almond Snack Bars
Ingredients:

- 1 1/2 cups rolled oats
- 1/2 cup dried cranberries
- 1/2 cup chopped almonds
- 1/2 cup almond butter
- 1/3 cup honey or maple syrup
- 1 teaspoon vanilla extract
- 1/4 teaspoon salt

Directions:

1. Preheat the oven to 350°F (175°C). Line an 8x8-inch baking dish with parchment paper.
2. In a large bowl, combine oats, dried cranberries, and chopped almonds.
3. In a separate bowl, mix together almond butter, honey or maple syrup, vanilla extract, and salt.

4. Pour the wet ingredients into the dry ingredients and mix until well combined.

5. Press the mixture into the prepared baking dish.

6. Bake for 20-25 minutes, or until set.

7. Let cool completely before cutting into bars.

Serving Size:

12 bars

Nutrition (per serving):

Calories: 180

Protein: 4g

Carbohydrates: 23g

Fat: 8g

Fiber: 4g

Sugar: 12g

4. Apple Cinnamon Snack Bars

Ingredients:

- 2 cups rolled oats
- 1/2 cup almond flour
- 1/2 cup unsweetened applesauce
- 1/2 cup chopped dried apples
- 1/2 cup honey or maple syrup
- 1 teaspoon cinnamon
- 1/2 teaspoon salt
- 1 teaspoon vanilla extract

Directions:

1. Preheat the oven to 350°F (175°C). Line an 8x8-inch baking dish with parchment paper.
2. In a large bowl, combine oats, almond flour, chopped dried apples, cinnamon, and salt.
3. In a separate bowl, mix together applesauce, honey or maple syrup, and vanilla extract.
4. Pour the wet ingredients into the dry ingredients and mix until well combined.
5. Press the mixture into the prepared baking dish.
6. Bake for 25-30 minutes, or until golden brown.
7. Let cool completely before cutting into bars.

Serving Size:

12 bars

Nutrition (per serving):

Calories: 170

Protein: 3g

Carbohydrates: 28g

Fat: 6g

Fiber: 4g

Sugar: 14g

5. Peanut Butter Banana Snack Bars

Ingredients:

- 2 cups rolled oats
- 1/2 cup peanut butter
- 1/2 cup mashed ripe banana
- 1/3 cup honey or maple syrup
- 1/4 cup ground flaxseed

- 1 teaspoon vanilla extract
- 1/4 teaspoon salt

Directions:

1. Preheat the oven to 350°F (175°C). Line an 8x8-inch baking dish with parchment paper.
2. In a large bowl, combine oats and ground flaxseed.
3. In a separate bowl, mix together peanut butter, mashed banana, honey or maple syrup, vanilla extract, and salt.
4. Pour the wet ingredients into the dry ingredients and mix until well combined.
5. Press the mixture into the prepared baking dish.
6. Bake for 25-30 minutes, or until golden brown.
7. Let cool completely before cutting into bars.

Serving Size:

12 bars

Nutrition (per serving):

Calories: 190

Protein: 5g

Carbohydrates: 25g

Fat: 8g

Fiber: 4g

Sugar: 12g

5.3 Hydrating Fruit and Veggie Snacks

1. Cucumber and Watermelon Salad

Ingredients:

- 2 cups cucumber, thinly sliced
- 2 cups watermelon, cubed
- 1/4 cup red onion, thinly sliced
- 2 tablespoons fresh mint, chopped
- 2 tablespoons feta cheese, crumbled
- 1 tablespoon olive oil
- 1 tablespoon lime juice
- Salt and pepper to taste

Directions:

1. In a large bowl, combine cucumber, watermelon, red onion, and mint.
2. Drizzle with olive oil and lime juice.
3. Toss gently to combine.
4. Top with feta cheese and season with salt and pepper.
5. Serve chilled.

Serving Size:

4 servings

Nutrition (per serving):

Calories: 90

Protein: 2g

Carbohydrates: 12g

Fat: 4g

Fiber: 1g

Sugar: 9g

2. Bell Pepper and Hummus Platter

Ingredients:

- 3 bell peppers (red, yellow, green), sliced
- 1 cup hummus
- 1 tablespoon olive oil
- 1 teaspoon paprika
- 1 teaspoon sesame seeds

Directions:

1. Arrange bell pepper slices on a serving platter.
2. Place hummus in a small bowl in the center of the platter.
3. Drizzle olive oil over the hummus and sprinkle with paprika and sesame seeds.
4. Serve immediately.

Serving Size:

4 servings

Nutrition (per serving):

Calories: 120

Protein: 3g

Carbohydrates: 15g

Fat: 6g

Fiber: 4g

Sugar: 6g

3. Pineapple and Cucumber Skewers

Ingredients:

- 2 cups pineapple, cubed
- 2 cups cucumber, cubed
- 1 tablespoon fresh mint, chopped
- 1 tablespoon lime juice

Directions:

1. Thread pineapple and cucumber cubes onto skewers, alternating between the two.
2. Place skewers on a serving platter.
3. Drizzle with lime juice and sprinkle with fresh mint.
4. Serve chilled.

Serving Size:

4 servings

Nutrition (per serving):

Calories: 70

Protein: 1g

Carbohydrates: 18g

Fat: 0g

Fiber: 2g

Sugar: 14g

4. Celery and Peanut Butter Sticks

Ingredients:

- 4 celery stalks, cut into sticks

- 1/2 cup peanut butter
- 2 tablespoons raisins

Directions:

1. Fill each celery stick with peanut butter.
2. Top with raisins.
3. Serve immediately.
4. Serving Size:

4 servings

Nutrition (per serving):

Calories: 150
Protein: 4g
Carbohydrates: 12g
Fat: 10g
Fiber: 3g
Sugar: 7g

5. Mixed Berry Salad

Ingredients:

- 1 cup strawberries, sliced
- 1 cup blueberries
- 1 cup raspberries
- 1 cup blackberries
- 1 tablespoon honey (optional)
- 1 tablespoon fresh mint, chopped

Directions:

1. In a large bowl, combine strawberries, blueberries, raspberries, and blackberries.
2. Drizzle with honey if using and sprinkle with fresh mint.
3. Toss gently to combine.
4. Serve immediately.

Serving Size:

4 servings

Nutrition (per serving):

Calories: 70

Protein: 1g

Carbohydrates: 18g

Fat: 0g

Fiber: 5g

Sugar: 12g

5.4 Easy-to-Make Smoothie Bowls

1. Berry Banana Smoothie Bowl

Ingredients:

- 1 banana, frozen
- 1 cup mixed berries (strawberries, blueberries, raspberries), frozen
- 1/2 cup Greek yogurt
- 1/2 cup almond milk
- 1 tablespoon honey (optional)

Toppings: fresh berries, granola, chia seeds

Directions:

1. In a blender, combine the frozen banana, mixed berries, Greek yogurt, almond milk, and honey.
2. Blend until smooth and creamy.
3. Pour the smoothie into a bowl.
4. Top with fresh berries, granola, and chia seeds.
5. Serve immediately.

Serving Size:

1 serving

Nutrition (per serving):

Calories: 350

Protein: 15g

Carbohydrates: 60g

Fat: 7g

Fiber: 12g

Sugar: 35g

2. Tropical Mango Smoothie Bowl

Ingredients:

- 1 mango, peeled and chopped
- 1 banana, frozen
- 1/2 cup pineapple chunks, frozen
- 1/2 cup coconut milk
- 1 tablespoon shredded coconut
- Toppings: sliced kiwi, chia seeds, granola

Directions:

1. In a blender, combine the mango, frozen banana, pineapple chunks, and coconut milk.
2. Blend until smooth and creamy.
3. Pour the smoothie into a bowl.
4. Top with sliced kiwi, chia seeds, and granola.
5. Serve immediately.

Serving Size:

1 serving

Nutrition (per serving):

Calories: 300

Protein: 4g

Carbohydrates: 68g

Fat: 6g

Fiber: 10g

Sugar: 44g

3. Green Goddess Smoothie Bowl

Ingredients:

- 1 banana, frozen
- 1/2 avocado
- 1 cup spinach
- 1/2 cup almond milk
- 1 tablespoon chia seeds
- 1 tablespoon honey (optional)
- Toppings: sliced banana, granola, pumpkin seeds

Directions:

1. In a blender, combine the frozen banana, avocado, spinach, almond milk, chia seeds, and honey.
2. Blend until smooth and creamy.
3. Pour the smoothie into a bowl.
4. Top with sliced banana, granola, and pumpkin seeds.
5. Serve immediately.

Serving Size:

1 serving

Nutrition (per serving):

Calories: 320

Protein: 6g

Carbohydrates: 45g

Fat: 14g

Fiber: 11g

Sugar: 20g

4. Peanut Butter Banana Smoothie Bowl

Ingredients:

- 1 banana, frozen
- 1/2 cup Greek yogurt
- 1/2 cup almond milk
- 2 tablespoons peanut butter
- 1 tablespoon honey (optional)
- Toppings: sliced banana, granola, cacao nibs

Directions:

1. In a blender, combine the frozen banana, Greek yogurt, almond milk, peanut butter, and honey.
2. Blend until smooth and creamy.
3. Pour the smoothie into a bowl.
4. Top with sliced banana, granola, and cacao nibs.
5. Serve immediately.

Serving Size:

1 serving

Nutrition (per serving):

Calories: 400

Protein: 18g

Carbohydrates: 50g

Fat: 16g

Fiber: 7g

Sugar: 28g

5. Acai Berry Smoothie Bowl

Ingredients:

- 1 packet frozen acai puree
- 1 banana, frozen
- 1/2 cup mixed berries (blueberries, raspberries), frozen
- 1/2 cup almond milk
- 1 tablespoon honey (optional)
- Toppings: sliced strawberries, granola, coconut flakes

Directions:

1. In a blender, combine the acai puree, frozen banana, mixed berries, almond milk, and honey.
2. Blend until smooth and creamy.
3. Pour the smoothie into a bowl.
4. Top with sliced strawberries, granola, and coconut flakes.
5. Serve immediately.
6. Serving Size:

1 serving

Nutrition (per serving):

Calories: 350
Protein: 6g
Carbohydrates: 70g
Fat: 8g
Fiber: 11g
Sugar: 35g

Chapter 6: Nourishing Dinners

6.1 Balanced One-Pot Meals

1. Chicken and Vegetable Stir-Fry

Ingredients:

- 1 lb chicken breast, cut into bite-sized pieces
- 2 tablespoons olive oil
- 1 bell pepper, sliced
- 1 zucchini, sliced
- 1 cup broccoli florets
- 1 cup snap peas
- 3 cloves garlic, minced
- 1/4 cup soy sauce (low sodium)
- 2 tablespoons hoisin sauce
- 1 tablespoon honey
- 1 teaspoon ginger, grated
- 1 cup cooked brown rice

Directions:

1. Heat 1 tablespoon of olive oil in a large skillet or wok over medium-high heat.
2. Add the chicken and cook until browned and cooked through, about 5-7 minutes. Remove from the skillet and set aside.
3. In the same skillet, add the remaining olive oil and garlic. Sauté for 1 minute.
4. Add the bell pepper, zucchini, broccoli, and snap peas. Stir-fry for 5-7 minutes until vegetables are tender-crisp.
5. Return the chicken to the skillet.

6. In a small bowl, mix soy sauce, hoisin sauce, honey, and ginger. Pour over the chicken and vegetables.

7. Stir well to coat and cook for an additional 2-3 minutes.

8. Serve over cooked brown rice.

Serving Size:

4 servings

Nutrition (per serving):

Calories: 380
Protein: 30g
Carbohydrates: 35g
Fat: 14g
Fiber: 5g
Sugar: 10g

2. Quinoa and Black Bean Skillet

Ingredients:

- 1 cup quinoa, rinsed
- 2 cups vegetable broth
- 1 can black beans, drained and rinsed
- 1 can diced tomatoes (14.5 oz)
- 1 cup corn kernels (fresh, frozen, or canned)
- 1 red bell pepper, chopped
- 1 small onion, chopped
- 2 cloves garlic, minced
- 1 teaspoon cumin
- 1 teaspoon chili powder
- 1/2 teaspoon paprika

- Salt and pepper to taste
- 1 avocado, sliced (for topping)
- Fresh cilantro, chopped (for garnish)

Directions:

1. In a large skillet, sauté onion and garlic over medium heat until softened.
2. Add the bell pepper and cook for another 2-3 minutes.
3. Stir in the quinoa, vegetable broth, black beans, diced tomatoes, corn, cumin, chili powder, paprika, salt, and pepper.
4. Bring to a boil, then reduce the heat to low. Cover and simmer for 20-25 minutes, or until the quinoa is cooked and the liquid is absorbed.
5. Fluff with a fork and serve topped with sliced avocado and fresh cilantro.

Serving Size:

4 servings

Nutrition (per serving):

Calories: 350
Protein: 12g
Carbohydrates: 60g
Fat: 8g
Fiber: 12g
Sugar: 6g

3. Beef and Barley Stew

Ingredients:

- 1 lb beef stew meat, cut into bite-sized pieces
- 2 tablespoons olive oil
- 1 onion, chopped

- 2 cloves garlic, minced
- 3 carrots, sliced
- 2 celery stalks, sliced
- 1 cup pearl barley
- 4 cups beef broth
- 1 can diced tomatoes (14.5 oz)
- 1 teaspoon thyme
- 1 teaspoon rosemary
- Salt and pepper to taste
- Fresh parsley, chopped (for garnish)

Directions:

1. Heat olive oil in a large pot over medium-high heat. Add the beef and brown on all sides.
2. Add the onion and garlic, sautéing until softened.
3. Stir in the carrots, celery, barley, beef broth, diced tomatoes, thyme, rosemary, salt, and pepper.
4. Bring to a boil, then reduce heat to low and simmer, covered, for 1 hour or until the beef and barley are tender.
5. Serve garnished with fresh parsley.

Serving Size:

6 servings

Nutrition (per serving):

Calories: 320

Protein: 20g

Carbohydrates: 40g

Fat: 10g

Fiber: 8g

Sugar: 6g

4. Mediterranean Chickpea Stew

Ingredients:

- 2 tablespoons olive oil
- 1 onion, chopped
- 3 cloves garlic, minced
- 2 cups baby spinach
- 1 can chickpeas (15 oz), drained and rinsed
- 1 can diced tomatoes (14.5 oz)
- 1 cup vegetable broth
- 1 teaspoon cumin
- 1 teaspoon paprika
- 1/2 teaspoon turmeric
- Salt and pepper to taste
- Fresh lemon juice (from 1 lemon)
- Fresh parsley, chopped (for garnish)

Directions:

1. Heat olive oil in a large pot over medium heat. Add the onion and garlic, sautéing until softened.
2. Stir in the cumin, paprika, turmeric, salt, and pepper.
3. Add the chickpeas, diced tomatoes, and vegetable broth. Bring to a boil.
4. Reduce heat to low and simmer for 20 minutes.
5. Stir in the baby spinach and cook until wilted.
6. Add fresh lemon juice and stir to combine.
7. Serve garnished with fresh parsley.

Serving Size:

4 servings

Nutrition (per serving):

Calories: 240
Protein: 7g
Carbohydrates: 30g
Fat: 10g
Fiber: 9g
Sugar: 6g

5. Shrimp and Vegetable Paella

Ingredients:

- 2 tablespoons olive oil
- 1 onion, chopped
- 3 cloves garlic, minced
- 1 bell pepper, chopped
- 1 cup green beans, chopped
- 1 cup cherry tomatoes, halved
- 1 cup arborio rice
- 2 cups chicken broth
- 1/2 teaspoon saffron threads (optional)
- 1 lb shrimp, peeled and deveined
- 1 lemon, cut into wedges
- Fresh parsley, chopped (for garnish)

Directions:

1. Heat olive oil in a large skillet or paella pan over medium heat. Add the onion and garlic, sautéing until softened.

2. Add the bell pepper, green beans, and cherry tomatoes. Cook for 5 minutes, stirring occasionally.
3. Stir in the arborio rice and cook for 2 minutes, toasting the rice.
4. Add the chicken broth and saffron threads (if using). Bring to a boil.
5. Reduce heat to low and simmer, covered, for 15 minutes.
6. Arrange the shrimp on top of the rice and cover again. Cook for an additional 5-7 minutes, or until the shrimp are pink and cooked through.
7. Serve with lemon wedges and garnish with fresh parsley.

Serving Size:

4 servings

Nutrition (per serving):

Calories: 380

Protein: 25g

Carbohydrates: 45g

Fat: 12g

Fiber: 4g

Sugar: 6g

6.2 Lean Protein Entrees

1. Baked Lemon Herb Chicken

Ingredients:

- 4 boneless, skinless chicken breasts
- 2 tablespoons olive oil
- 2 cloves garlic, minced
- 1 lemon, juiced and zested
- 1 teaspoon dried thyme
- 1 teaspoon dried rosemary
- Salt and pepper to taste
- Fresh parsley, chopped (for garnish)

Directions:

1. Preheat the oven to 400°F (200°C). Grease a baking dish with olive oil.
2. In a small bowl, mix olive oil, garlic, lemon juice and zest, thyme, rosemary, salt, and pepper.
3. Place chicken breasts in the baking dish and pour the lemon herb mixture over them, turning to coat evenly.
4. Bake for 20-25 minutes, or until chicken is cooked through and juices run clear.
5. Garnish with fresh parsley before serving.

Serving Size:

4 servings

Nutrition (per serving):

Calories: 250

Protein: 30g

Carbohydrates: 2g

Fat: 12g

Fiber: 0g

Sugar: 0g

2. Grilled Lemon Garlic Shrimp

Ingredients:

- 1 lb shrimp, peeled and deveined
- 2 tablespoons olive oil
- 3 cloves garlic, minced
- 1 lemon, juiced and zested
- 1 teaspoon dried oregano
- Salt and pepper to taste
- Fresh parsley, chopped (for garnish)

Directions:

1. Preheat grill to medium-high heat.
2. In a bowl, combine olive oil, garlic, lemon juice and zest, oregano, salt, and pepper.
3. Add shrimp to the bowl and toss to coat evenly.
4. Thread shrimp onto skewers or use a grill basket.
5. Grill shrimp for 2-3 minutes per side, until pink and opaque.
6. Garnish with fresh parsley before serving.

Serving Size:

4 servings

Nutrition (per serving):

Calories: 180

Protein: 25g

Carbohydrates: 2g

Fat: 8g

Fiber: 0g

Sugar: 0g

3. Baked Salmon with Dill Sauce

Ingredients:

- 4 salmon fillets
- 2 tablespoons olive oil
- Salt and pepper to taste
- 1 lemon, sliced
- Fresh dill, chopped

Dill Sauce:

- 1/2 cup plain Greek yogurt
- 1 tablespoon fresh dill, chopped
- 1 tablespoon lemon juice
- Salt and pepper to taste

Directions:

1. Preheat the oven to 400°F (200°C). Grease a baking dish with olive oil.
2. Place salmon fillets in the baking dish and drizzle with olive oil. Season with salt and pepper.
3. Arrange lemon slices on top of the salmon.
4. Bake for 12-15 minutes, or until salmon flakes easily with a fork.
5. While salmon is baking, prepare the dill sauce by mixing Greek yogurt, fresh dill, lemon juice, salt, and pepper in a bowl.
6. Serve baked salmon with dill sauce on the side, garnished with additional fresh dill.

Serving Size:

4 servings

Nutrition (per serving):

Calories: 300

Protein: 30g

Carbohydrates: 3g

Fat: 18g

Fiber: 0g

Sugar: 1g

4. Turkey and Vegetable Stir-Fry

Ingredients:

- 1 lb turkey breast, cut into strips
- 2 tablespoons soy sauce (low sodium)
- 1 tablespoon olive oil
- 2 cloves garlic, minced
- 1 onion, sliced
- 1 bell pepper, sliced
- 1 cup snow peas
- 1 cup broccoli florets
- 1 teaspoon ginger, grated
- Salt and pepper to taste
- Cooked brown rice or quinoa (optional, for serving)

Directions:

1. In a bowl, marinate turkey strips in soy sauce for 10-15 minutes.
2. Heat olive oil in a large skillet or wok over medium-high heat.

3. Add garlic and onion, sautéing until softened.

4. Add marinated turkey to the skillet, cooking until browned and cooked through.

5. Stir in bell pepper, snow peas, broccoli, ginger, salt, and pepper. Stir-fry for 5-7 minutes, until vegetables are tender-crisp.

6. Serve turkey and vegetable stir-fry hot, over cooked brown rice or quinoa if desired.

Serving Size:

4 servings

Nutrition (per serving):

Calories: 280

Protein: 30g

Carbohydrates: 10g

Fat: 12g

Fiber: 3g

Sugar: 4g

5. Lemon Garlic Baked Tofu

Ingredients:

- 1 block tofu, extra firm, drained and pressed
- 2 tablespoons olive oil
- 2 cloves garlic, minced
- 1 lemon, juiced and zested
- 1 teaspoon dried thyme
- Salt and pepper to taste
- Fresh parsley, chopped (for garnish)

Directions:

1. Preheat the oven to 400°F (200°C). Grease a baking dish with olive oil.
2. Cut tofu into cubes and place in the baking dish.
3. In a bowl, combine olive oil, garlic, lemon juice and zest, thyme, salt, and pepper.
4. Pour the lemon garlic mixture over the tofu, tossing gently to coat.
5. Bake for 25-30 minutes, flipping halfway through, until tofu is golden and crispy.
6. Garnish with fresh parsley before serving.

Serving Size:

4 servings

Nutrition (per serving):

Calories: 200

Protein: 14g

Carbohydrates: 6g

Fat: 14g

Fiber: 1g

Sugar: 1g

6.3 Wholesome Grain and Vegetable Sides

1. Quinoa and Roasted Vegetables

Ingredients:

- 1 cup quinoa, rinsed
- 2 cups vegetable broth
- 1 red bell pepper, chopped
- 1 yellow bell pepper, chopped
- 1 zucchini, chopped
- 1 red onion, chopped
- 2 tablespoons olive oil
- 1 teaspoon dried thyme
- Salt and pepper to taste
- Fresh parsley, chopped (for garnish)

Directions:

1. Preheat the oven to 400°F (200°C).
2. In a large bowl, toss chopped bell peppers, zucchini, and red onion with olive oil, thyme, salt, and pepper.
3. Spread vegetables evenly on a baking sheet and roast for 20-25 minutes, or until tender and lightly browned, stirring halfway through.
4. In a saucepan, bring vegetable broth to a boil. Add quinoa, reduce heat to low, cover, and simmer for 15 minutes or until quinoa is cooked and liquid is absorbed.
5. Fluff quinoa with a fork and stir in roasted vegetables.
6. Garnish with fresh parsley before serving.

Serving Size:

4 servings

Nutrition (per serving):

Calories: 250
Protein: 7g
Carbohydrates: 35g
Fat: 10g
Fiber: 5g
Sugar: 5g

2. Lemon Garlic Brown Rice

Ingredients:

- 1 cup brown rice, rinsed
- 2 cups vegetable broth
- 2 tablespoons olive oil
- 2 cloves garlic, minced
- 1 lemon, juiced and zested
- Salt and pepper to taste
- Fresh parsley, chopped (for garnish)

Directions:

1. In a saucepan, heat olive oil over medium heat. Add garlic and sauté until fragrant.
2. Stir in brown rice and cook for 1-2 minutes, toasting the rice.
3. Add vegetable broth, lemon juice and zest, salt, and pepper. Bring to a boil.
4. Reduce heat to low, cover, and simmer for 40-45 minutes, or until rice is tender and liquid is absorbed.
5. Fluff rice with a fork and garnish with fresh parsley before serving.

Serving Size:

4 servings

Nutrition (per serving):

Calories: 220
Protein: 5g
Carbohydrates: 35g
Fat: 7g
Fiber: 3g
Sugar: 1g

3. Garlic Parmesan Roasted Brussels Sprouts

Ingredients:

- 1 lb Brussels sprouts, trimmed and halved
- 2 tablespoons olive oil
- 2 cloves garlic, minced
- 1/4 cup grated Parmesan cheese
- Salt and pepper to taste
- Lemon wedges (for serving)

Directions:

1. Preheat the oven to 400°F (200°C).
2. In a large bowl, toss Brussels sprouts with olive oil, garlic, Parmesan cheese, salt, and pepper.
3. Spread Brussels sprouts evenly on a baking sheet.
4. Roast for 20-25 minutes, or until Brussels sprouts are golden and crispy, stirring halfway through.
5. Serve with lemon wedges for squeezing over the roasted Brussels sprouts.

Serving Size:

4 servings

Nutrition (per serving):

Calories: 150
Protein: 6g
Carbohydrates: 12g
Fat: 10g
Fiber: 5g
Sugar: 3g

4. Mediterranean Couscous Salad

Ingredients:

- 1 cup couscous, uncooked
- 1 1/4 cups vegetable broth
- 1 cucumber, diced
- 1 cup cherry tomatoes, halved
- 1/4 cup Kalamata olives, sliced
- 1/4 cup red onion, finely chopped
- 1/4 cup feta cheese, crumbled
- 2 tablespoons olive oil
- 1 tablespoon lemon juice
- 1 teaspoon dried oregano
- Salt and pepper to taste
- Fresh parsley, chopped (for garnish)

Directions:

1. In a saucepan, bring vegetable broth to a boil. Add couscous, cover, and remove from heat. Let stand for 5 minutes, then fluff with a fork.

2. In a large bowl, combine cooked couscous, cucumber, cherry tomatoes, Kalamata olives, red onion, and feta cheese.

3. In a small bowl, whisk together olive oil, lemon juice, dried oregano, salt, and pepper.

4. Pour dressing over couscous salad and toss to coat evenly.

5. Garnish with fresh parsley before serving.

Serving Size:

4 servings

Nutrition (per serving):

Calories: 280

Protein: 8g

Carbohydrates: 38g

Fat: 10g

Fiber: 4g

Sugar: 3g

5. Herb Roasted Sweet Potatoes

Ingredients:

- 2 large sweet potatoes, peeled and diced
- 2 tablespoons olive oil
- 1 teaspoon dried thyme
- 1 teaspoon dried rosemary
- Salt and pepper to taste
- Fresh parsley, chopped (for garnish)

Directions:

1. Preheat the oven to 400°F (200°C).

2. In a large bowl, toss sweet potatoes with olive oil, thyme, rosemary, salt, and pepper.

3. Spread sweet potatoes evenly on a baking sheet.

4. Roast for 30-35 minutes, or until sweet potatoes are tender and caramelized, stirring halfway through.

5. Garnish with fresh parsley before serving.

Serving Size:

4 servings

Nutrition (per serving):

Calories: 180

Protein: 2g

Carbohydrates: 27g

Fat: 8g

Fiber: 4g

Sugar: 6g

6.4 Flavorful and Hydrating Stews

1. Chicken and Vegetable Quinoa Stew

Ingredients:

- 1 lb chicken breast, cut into bite-sized pieces
- 1 tablespoon olive oil
- 1 onion, chopped
- 2 cloves garlic, minced
- 2 carrots, sliced
- 2 celery stalks, sliced
- 1 bell pepper, chopped
- 1 cup quinoa, rinsed
- 4 cups chicken broth
- 1 can diced tomatoes (14.5 oz)
- 1 teaspoon dried thyme
- Salt and pepper to taste
- Fresh parsley, chopped (for garnish)

Directions:

1. In a large pot, heat olive oil over medium-high heat. Add chicken and cook until browned.
2. Add onion and garlic, sautéing until softened.
3. Stir in carrots, celery, bell pepper, and quinoa. Cook for 2-3 minutes.
4. Pour in chicken broth and diced tomatoes. Add dried thyme, salt, and pepper.
5. Bring to a boil, then reduce heat to low. Cover and simmer for 20-25 minutes, or until quinoa is cooked and vegetables are tender.
6. Serve hot, garnished with fresh parsley.

Serving Size:

4 servings

Nutrition (per serving):

Calories: 350

Protein: 30g

Carbohydrates: 40g

Fat: 8g

Fiber: 6g

Sugar: 6g

2. Lentil and Vegetable Stew

Ingredients:

- 1 cup green lentils, rinsed
- 4 cups vegetable broth
- 1 onion, chopped
- 2 cloves garlic, minced
- 2 carrots, sliced
- 2 celery stalks, sliced
- 1 sweet potato, peeled and diced
- 1 can diced tomatoes (14.5 oz)
- 1 teaspoon ground cumin
- 1 teaspoon smoked paprika
- Salt and pepper to taste
- Fresh cilantro, chopped (for garnish)

Directions:

1. In a large pot, combine green lentils and vegetable broth. Bring to a boil.
2. Reduce heat to low, cover, and simmer for 15 minutes.

3. In a skillet, heat olive oil over medium heat. Add onion and garlic, sautéing until softened.

4. Add carrots, celery, and sweet potato to the skillet. Cook for 5-7 minutes, until vegetables begin to soften.

5. Transfer vegetable mixture to the pot with lentils. Add diced tomatoes, cumin, smoked paprika, salt, and pepper.

6. Cover and simmer for an additional 20-25 minutes, or until lentils and vegetables are tender.

7. Serve hot, garnished with fresh cilantro.

Serving Size:

4 servings

Nutrition (per serving):

Calories: 320

Protein: 18g

Carbohydrates: 60g

Fat: 2g

Fiber: 18g

Sugar: 10g

3. Beef and Barley Vegetable Soup

Ingredients:

- 1 lb beef stew meat, cut into bite-sized pieces
- 1 tablespoon olive oil
- 1 onion, chopped
- 2 cloves garlic, minced
- 2 carrots, sliced
- 2 celery stalks, sliced

- 1 cup pearl barley
- 6 cups beef broth
- 1 can diced tomatoes (14.5 oz)
- 1 teaspoon dried thyme
- Salt and pepper to taste
- Fresh parsley, chopped (for garnish)

Directions:

1. In a large pot, heat olive oil over medium-high heat. Add beef and cook until browned.
2. Add onion and garlic, sautéing until softened.
3. Stir in carrots, celery, and pearl barley. Cook for 2-3 minutes.
4. Pour in beef broth and diced tomatoes. Add dried thyme, salt, and pepper.
5. Bring to a boil, then reduce heat to low. Cover and simmer for 1 hour, or until beef and barley are tender.
6. Serve hot, garnished with fresh parsley.

Serving Size:

6 servings

Nutrition (per serving):

Calories: 380

Protein: 28g

Carbohydrates: 45g

Fat: 10g

Fiber: 10g

Sugar: 6g

4. Moroccan Chickpea Stew

Ingredients:

- 2 tablespoons olive oil
- 1 onion, chopped
- 3 cloves garlic, minced
- 1 carrot, diced
- 1 bell pepper, diced
- 1 zucchini, diced
- 1 teaspoon ground cumin
- 1 teaspoon ground coriander
- 1/2 teaspoon cinnamon
- 1 can chickpeas (15 oz), drained and rinsed
- 1 can diced tomatoes (14.5 oz)
- 4 cups vegetable broth
- Salt and pepper to taste
- Fresh cilantro, chopped (for garnish)

Directions:

1. In a large pot, heat olive oil over medium heat. Add onion and garlic, sautéing until softened.
2. Stir in carrot, bell pepper, and zucchini. Cook for 5-7 minutes, until vegetables begin to soften.
3. Add ground cumin, ground coriander, and cinnamon to the pot. Stir to coat vegetables.
4. Add chickpeas, diced tomatoes, and vegetable broth. Season with salt and pepper.
5. Bring to a boil, then reduce heat to low. Cover and simmer for 20-25 minutes, or until vegetables are tender.
6. Serve hot, garnished with fresh cilantro.

Serving Size:

4 servings

Nutrition (per serving):

Calories: 280
Protein: 10g
Carbohydrates: 40g
Fat: 10g
Fiber: 10g
Sugar: 8g

5. Thai Coconut Curry Vegetable Soup
Ingredients:

- 1 tablespoon olive oil
- 1 onion, chopped
- 3 cloves garlic, minced
- 1 tablespoon fresh ginger, grated
- 2 tablespoons Thai red curry paste
- 1 sweet potato, peeled and diced
- 1 red bell pepper, diced
- 1 zucchini, diced
- 1 can coconut milk (13.5 oz)
- 4 cups vegetable broth
- 1 tablespoon soy sauce (low sodium)
- Juice of 1 lime
- Salt and pepper to taste
- Fresh cilantro, chopped (for garnish)

Directions:

1. In a large pot, heat olive oil over medium heat. Add onion, garlic, and ginger, sautéing until softened.
2. Stir in Thai red curry paste and cook for 1 minute, until fragrant.
3. Add sweet potato, red bell pepper, zucchini, coconut milk, vegetable broth, and soy sauce. Bring to a boil.
4. Reduce heat to low, cover, and simmer for 20-25 minutes, or until vegetables are tender.
5. Stir in lime juice and season with salt and pepper.
6. Serve hot, garnished with fresh cilantro.

Serving Size:

4 servings

Nutrition (per serving):

Calories: 320

Protein: 6g

Carbohydrates: 30g

Fat: 22g

Fiber: 6g

Sugar: 8g

Chapter 7: Delicious and Healthy Desserts

7.1 Low-Sugar Treats

1. Dark Chocolate Avocado Mousse

Ingredients:

- 2 ripe avocados
- 1/4 cup cocoa powder (unsweetened)
- 1/4 cup honey or maple syrup
- 1 teaspoon vanilla extract
- Pinch of salt
- Fresh berries (for garnish)

Directions:

1. Scoop the flesh of avocados into a food processor or blender.
2. Add cocoa powder, honey or maple syrup, vanilla extract, and a pinch of salt.
3. Blend until smooth and creamy, scraping down the sides as needed.
4. Divide into serving dishes and refrigerate for at least 30 minutes.
5. Serve chilled, garnished with fresh berries.

Serving Size:

4 servings

Nutrition (per serving):

Calories: 200

Protein: 3g

Carbohydrates: 22g

Fat: 13g

Fiber: 6g

Sugar: 12g

2. Banana Oatmeal Cookies

Ingredients:

- 2 ripe bananas, mashed
- 1 cup rolled oats
- 1/4 cup chopped nuts (optional)
- 1/4 cup chocolate chips (optional)
- 1 teaspoon vanilla extract
- Pinch of cinnamon (optional)

Directions:

1. Preheat the oven to 350°F (175°C). Line a baking sheet with parchment paper.
2. In a bowl, combine mashed bananas, rolled oats, nuts (if using), chocolate chips (if using), vanilla extract, and cinnamon (if using).
3. Drop spoonfuls of the mixture onto the prepared baking sheet, shaping into cookies.
4. Bake for 15-20 minutes, or until cookies are golden brown.
5. Allow to cool on a wire rack before serving.

Serving Size:

12 cookies

Nutrition (per serving, 1 cookie):

Calories: 80

Protein: 1g

Carbohydratcs: 15g

Fat: 2g

Fiber: 1g
Sugar: 5g

3. Greek Yogurt Berry Popsicles

Ingredients:

- 1 cup Greek yogurt (plain, unsweetened)
- 1 cup mixed berries (such as strawberries, blueberries, raspberries)
- 2 tablespoons honey or maple syrup (optional)

Directions:

1. In a blender, combine Greek yogurt, mixed berries, and honey or maple syrup (if using).
2. Blend until smooth.
3. Pour mixture into popsicle molds.
4. Insert popsicle sticks and freeze for at least 4 hours, or until solid.
5. Run molds under warm water to release popsicles before serving.

Serving Size:
6 popsicles

Nutrition (per serving, 1 popsicle):

Calories: 50
Protein: 3g
Carbohydrates: 8g
Fat: 1g
Fiber: 1g
Sugar: 7g

4. Almond Butter Energy Bites

Ingredients:

- 1 cup rolled oats
- 1/2 cup almond butter (unsweetened)
- 1/4 cup honey or maple syrup
- 1/4 cup ground flaxseed
- 1/4 cup mini chocolate chips (optional)
- 1 teaspoon vanilla extract

Directions:

1. In a bowl, combine rolled oats, almond butter, honey or maple syrup, ground flaxseed, chocolate chips (if using), and vanilla extract.
2. Stir until well combined.
3. Roll mixture into small balls using your hands.
4. Place energy bites on a baking sheet lined with parchment paper.
5. Refrigerate for at least 30 minutes before serving.

Serving Size:

16 energy bites

Nutrition (per serving, 1 energy bite):

Calories: 100

Protein: 3g

Carbohydrates: 11g

Fat: 5g

Fiber: 2g

Sugar: 5g

5. Coconut Chia Seed Pudding

Ingredients:

- 1/4 cup chia seeds
- 1 cup coconut milk (unsweetened)
- 1 tablespoon honey or maple syrup
- 1/2 teaspoon vanilla extract
- Fresh berries or shredded coconut (for garnish)

Directions:

1. In a bowl, combine chia seeds, coconut milk, honey or maple syrup, and vanilla extract.
2. Whisk until well combined.
3. Cover and refrigerate for at least 2 hours, or overnight, stirring occasionally.
4. Serve chilled, topped with fresh berries or shredded coconut.

Serving Size:

2 servings

Nutrition (per serving):

Calories: 220

Protein: 4g

Carbohydrates: 20g

Fat: 14g

Fiber: 10g

Sugar: 8g

7.2 Hydrating Gelatin Desserts

1. Mixed Berry Gelatin Cups

Ingredients:

- 1 cup mixed berries (such as strawberries, blueberries, raspberries)
- 2 tablespoons honey or maple syrup
- 1 packet (about 2 1/2 teaspoons) unflavored gelatin
- 1 cup water
- Fresh mint leaves (for garnish)

Directions:

1. In a small saucepan, combine the mixed berries and honey or maple syrup. Cook over medium heat until the berries soften and release their juices, about 5-7 minutes.
2. In a separate bowl, sprinkle the gelatin over 1/4 cup of water and let it bloom for 5 minutes.
3. Add the remaining 3/4 cup of water to the saucepan with the berries and bring to a simmer.
4. Pour the hot berry mixture over the bloomed gelatin, stirring until the gelatin completely dissolves.
5. Divide the mixture into individual serving cups or molds.
6. Refrigerate for at least 2 hours, or until set.
7. Garnish with fresh mint leaves before serving.

Serving Size:

4 servings

Nutrition (per serving):

Calories: 50

Protein: 1g

Carbohydrates: 12g

Fat: 0g

Fiber: 2g

Sugar: 9g

2. Tropical Coconut Gelatin Squares

Ingredients:

- 1 can (13.5 oz) coconut milk
- 1/4 cup honey or agave syrup
- 1 packet (about 2 1/2 teaspoons) unflavored gelatin
- 1/2 cup pineapple juice
- 1/2 cup mango chunks (fresh or frozen)
- Shredded coconut (for garnish)

Directions:

1. In a saucepan, heat the coconut milk and honey or agave syrup over medium heat until warm but not boiling.
2. In a separate bowl, sprinkle the gelatin over 1/4 cup of pineapple juice and let it bloom for 5 minutes.
3. Add the remaining 1/4 cup of pineapple juice to the warm coconut milk mixture and stir well.
4. Pour the warm coconut milk mixture over the bloomed gelatin, stirring until the gelatin completely dissolves.
5. Stir in the mango chunks.
6. Pour the mixture into a square baking dish.
7. Refrigerate for at least 3 hours, or until set.
8. Cut into squares and garnish with shredded coconut before serving.

Serving Size:

12 squares

Nutrition (per serving, 1 square):

Calories: 70

Protein: 1g

Carbohydrates: 8g

Fat: 4g

Fiber: 0g

Sugar: 7g

3. Lemon Ginger Gelatin Cups

Ingredients:

- 1 cup water
- 1/4 cup honey or maple syrup
- 1 packet (about 2 1/2 teaspoons) unflavored gelatin
- 1/2 cup lemon juice
- 1 tablespoon grated fresh ginger
- Lemon zest (for garnish)

Directions:

1. In a small saucepan, combine the water and honey or maple syrup. Heat over medium heat until warm.
2. In a separate bowl, sprinkle the gelatin over 1/4 cup of lemon juice and let it bloom for 5 minutes.
3. Add the remaining 1/4 cup of lemon juice and grated ginger to the warm water mixture, stirring well.

4. Pour the hot lemon-ginger mixture over the bloomed gelatin, stirring until the gelatin completely dissolves.

5. Divide the mixture into individual serving cups or molds.

6. Refrigerate for at least 2 hours, or until set.

7. Garnish with lemon zest before serving.

Serving Size:

4 servings

Nutrition (per serving):

Calories: 40
Protein: 1g
Carbohydrates: 10g
Fat: 0g
Fiber: 0g
Sugar: 9g

4. Watermelon Lime Gelatin Cups

Ingredients:

- 2 cups watermelon juice (strained)
- Juice of 2 limes
- 2 tablespoons honey or agave syrup
- 1 packet (about 2 1/2 teaspoons) unflavored gelatin
- Fresh mint leaves (for garnish)

Directions:

1. In a small saucepan, heat the watermelon juice, lime juice, and honey or agave syrup over medium heat until warm.

2. In a separate bowl, sprinkle the gelatin over 1/4 cup of the warm
   watermelon-lime mixture and let it bloom for 5 minutes.
3. Add the bloomed gelatin back into the saucepan with the remaining
   watermelon-lime mixture, stirring until the gelatin completely dissolves.
4. Divide the mixture into individual serving cups or molds.
5. Refrigerate for at least 3 hours, or until set.
6. Garnish with fresh mint leaves before serving.

Serving Size:

4 servings

Nutrition (per serving):

Calories: 60

Protein: 2g

Carbohydrates: 14g

Fat: 0g

Fiber: 0g

Sugar: 12g

5. Herbal Tea Jelly with Mixed Berries

Ingredients:

- 2 cups brewed herbal tea (such as chamomile or berry-flavored)
- 1/4 cup honey or maple syrup
- 1 packet (about 2 1/2 teaspoons) unflavored gelatin
- 1 cup mixed berries (such as strawberries, blueberries)
- Fresh mint leaves (for garnish)

Directions:

1. In a saucepan, heat the brewed herbal tea and honey or maple syrup over medium heat until warm.
2. In a separate bowl, sprinkle the gelatin over 1/4 cup of the warm herbal tea mixture and let it bloom for 5 minutes.
3. Add the bloomed gelatin back into the saucepan with the remaining herbal tea mixture, stirring until the gelatin completely dissolves.
4. Divide the mixed berries into individual serving cups or molds.
5. Pour the herbal tea mixture over the berries.
6. Refrigerate for at least 4 hours, or until set.
7. Garnish with fresh mint leaves before serving.

Serving Size:

4 servings

Nutrition (per serving):

Calories: 50
Protein: 2g
Carbohydrates: 12g
Fat: 0g
Fiber: 1g
Sugar: 9g

7.3 Protein-Rich Puddings and Mousses

1. Chocolate Avocado Protein Mousse

Ingredients:

- 2 ripe avocados
- 1/4 cup cocoa powder (unsweetened)
- 1/4 cup honey or maple syrup
- 1 scoop chocolate protein powder
- 1 teaspoon vanilla extract
- Pinch of salt
- Fresh berries (for garnish)

Directions:

1. Scoop the flesh of avocados into a food processor or blender.
2. Add cocoa powder, honey or maple syrup, chocolate protein powder, vanilla extract, and a pinch of salt.
3. Blend until smooth and creamy, scraping down the sides as needed.
4. Divide into serving dishes and refrigerate for at least 30 minutes.
5. Serve chilled, garnished with fresh berries.

Serving Size:

4 servings

Nutrition (per serving):

Calories: 250

Protein: 10g

Carbohydrates: 30g

Fat: 14g

Fiber: 8g

Sugar: 18g

2. Greek Yogurt Chia Seed Pudding

Ingredients:

- 1 cup Greek yogurt (plain, unsweetened)
- 1/4 cup chia seeds
- 1 cup almond milk (unsweetened)
- 2 tablespoons honey or maple syrup
- 1 teaspoon vanilla extract
- Fresh berries (for garnish)

Directions:

1. In a bowl, combine Greek yogurt, chia seeds, almond milk, honey or maple syrup, and vanilla extract.
2. Stir until well combined.
3. Cover and refrigerate for at least 2 hours, or overnight, stirring occasionally.
4. Serve chilled, topped with fresh berries.

Serving Size:

2 servings

Nutrition (per serving):

Calories: 220
Protein: 15g
Carbohydrates: 25g
Fat: 8g
Fiber: 10g
Sugar: 15g

3. Vanilla Bean Cottage Cheese Pudding

Ingredients:

- 2 cups cottage cheese (low-fat)
- 1/4 cup honey or agave syrup
- 1 vanilla bean (seeds scraped out) or 1 tablespoon vanilla extract
- Fresh fruit slices (for garnish)

Directions:

1. In a food processor or blender, blend cottage cheese, honey or agave syrup, and vanilla bean seeds (or vanilla extract) until smooth.
2. Divide into serving bowls or cups.
3. Refrigerate for at least 1 hour before serving.
4. Garnish with fresh fruit slices before serving.

Serving Size:

4 servings

Nutrition (per serving):

Calories: 180

Protein: 15g

Carbohydrates: 20g

Fat: 5g

Fiber: 1g

Sugar: 15g

4. Chocolate Peanut Butter Protein Pudding

Ingredients:

- 1 cup plain Greek yogurt

- 2 tablespoons cocoa powder (unsweetened)
- 2 tablespoons peanut butter (unsweetened)
- 2 tablespoons honey or maple syrup
- 1 scoop chocolate protein powder
- Fresh banana slices (for garnish)

Directions:

1. In a bowl, whisk together Greek yogurt, cocoa powder, peanut butter, honey or maple syrup, and chocolate protein powder until smooth.
2. Divide into serving dishes.
3. Refrigerate for at least 1 hour before serving.
4. Garnish with fresh banana slices before serving.

Serving Size:

2 servings

Nutrition (per serving):

Calories: 280

Protein: 25g

Carbohydrates: 25g

Fat: 10g

Fiber: 4g

Sugar: 18g

5. Almond Tofu Mousse

Ingredients:

- 1 package (14 oz) soft tofu
- 1/4 cup almond butter (unsweetened)
- 2 tablespoons honey or agave syrup

- 1 teaspoon almond extract
- Sliced almonds (for garnish)

Directions:

1. In a food processor or blender, blend soft tofu, almond butter, honey or agave syrup, and almond extract until smooth.
2. Divide into serving bowls or cups.
3. Refrigerate for at least 1 hour before serving.
4. Garnish with sliced almonds before serving.

Serving Size:

4 servings

Nutrition (per serving):

Calories: 200

Protein: 12g

Carbohydrates: 15g

Fat: 12g

Fiber: 3g

Sugar: 10g

7.4 Fresh and Fruity Desserts

1. Mixed Berry Parfait

Ingredients:

- 1 cup mixed berries (such as strawberries, blueberries, raspberries)
- 1 cup Greek yogurt (plain, unsweetened)
- 1/2 cup granola (optional)
- Honey or maple syrup (optional, for sweetness)
- Fresh mint leaves (for garnish)

Directions:

1. Wash and prepare the mixed berries as needed.
2. In serving glasses or bowls, layer Greek yogurt, mixed berries, and granola (if using).
3. Repeat the layers until the glasses are filled, ending with a layer of berries on top.
4. Drizzle with honey or maple syrup for extra sweetness if desired.
5. Garnish with fresh mint leaves before serving.

Serving Size:

2 servings

Nutrition (per serving):

Calories: 200

Protein: 12g

Carbohydrates: 30g

Fat: 4g

Fiber: 6g

Sugar: 16g

2. Tropical Fruit Salad with Lime Mint Dressing

Ingredients:

- 2 cups mixed tropical fruits (such as pineapple, mango, kiwi)
- Juice of 1 lime
- 2 tablespoons honey or agave syrup
- Fresh mint leaves (chopped, for dressing and garnish)

Directions:

1. Prepare and dice the mixed tropical fruits into bite-sized pieces.
2. In a small bowl, whisk together lime juice, honey or agave syrup, and chopped mint leaves.
3. Pour the dressing over the mixed fruits and toss gently to coat.
4. Refrigerate for at least 30 minutes before serving.
5. Garnish with additional mint leaves before serving.

Serving Size:

2 servings

Nutrition (per serving):

Calories: 150

Protein: 2g

Carbohydrates: 38g

Fat: 0g

Fiber: 5g

Sugar: 30g

3. Lemon Blueberry Frozen Yogurt

Ingredients:

- 2 cups frozen blueberries
- 1 cup Greek yogurt (plain, unsweetened)
- Zest and juice of 1 lemon
- 2 tablespoons honey or maple syrup

Directions:

1. In a blender or food processor, combine frozen blueberries, Greek yogurt, lemon zest, lemon juice, and honey or maple syrup.
2. Blend until smooth and creamy, scraping down the sides as needed.
3. Transfer to a container and freeze for at least 2 hours, stirring occasionally, until firm.
4. Serve chilled, optionally garnished with fresh blueberries.

Serving Size:

4 servings

Nutrition (per serving):

Calories: 120

Protein: 5g

Carbohydrates: 25g

Fat: 1g

Fiber: 4g

Sugar: 19g

4. Kiwi Coconut Popsicles

Ingredients:

- 4 kiwis (peeled and sliced)
- 1 cup coconut water
- 2 tablespoons honey or agave syrup
- Fresh kiwi slices (for garnish)

Directions:

1. In a blender, combine kiwi slices, coconut water, and honey or agave syrup.
2. Blend until smooth.
3. Pour the mixture into popsicle molds.
4. Insert popsicle sticks and freeze for at least 4 hours, or until solid.
5. Run molds under warm water to release popsicles before serving.
6. Garnish with fresh kiwi slices before serving.

Serving Size:

4 popsicles

Nutrition (per serving, 1 popsicle):

Calories: 50

Protein: 1g

Carbohydrates: 12g

Fat: 0g

Fiber: 2g

Sugar: 9g

5. Pineapple Mango Sorbet

Ingredients:

- 2 cups frozen pineapple chunks
- 1 cup frozen mango chunks
- Juice of 1 lime
- 2 tablespoons honey or agave syrup

Directions:

1. In a blender or food processor, combine frozen pineapple chunks, frozen mango chunks, lime juice, and honey or agave syrup.
2. Blend until smooth and creamy, scraping down the sides as needed.
3. Transfer to a container and freeze for at least 2 hours, stirring occasionally, until firm.
4. Serve chilled, optionally garnished with fresh mint leaves.

Serving Size:

4 servings

Nutrition (per serving):

Calories: 120

Protein: 1g

Carbohydrates: 32g

Fat: 0g

Fiber: 3g

Sugar: 27g

Chapter 8: Hydrating Beverages

8.1 Electrolyte-Rich Drinks

1. Citrus Electrolyte Drink

Ingredients:

- 1 cup orange juice (freshly squeezed)
- 1/2 cup lemon juice (freshly squeezed)
- 2 cups coconut water
- 1/4 teaspoon sea salt
- 2 tablespoons honey or maple syrup
- 1 cup cold water

Directions:

1. In a large pitcher, combine the orange juice, lemon juice, coconut water, sea salt, and honey or maple syrup.
2. Stir well until the honey or maple syrup and salt are fully dissolved.
3. Add the cold water and stir again.
4. Chill in the refrigerator for at least 1 hour before serving.
5. Serve over ice if desired.

Serving Size:

4 servings

Nutrition (per serving):

Calories: 80

Protein: 1g

Carbohydrates: 21g

Fat: 0g

Fiber: 0g

Sugar: 18g

2. Watermelon Electrolyte Drink

Ingredients:

- 2 cups watermelon (diced)
- 1/2 cup coconut water
- Juice of 1 lime
- 1/4 teaspoon sea salt
- 1 tablespoon honey or agave syrup
- 1 cup cold water

Directions:

1. In a blender, combine the watermelon, coconut water, lime juice, sea salt, and honey or agave syrup.
2. Blend until smooth.
3. Strain the mixture through a fine-mesh sieve into a pitcher to remove any pulp.
4. Add the cold water and stir well.
5. Chill in the refrigerator for at least 1 hour before serving.
6. Serve over ice if desired.

Serving Size:

4 servings

Nutrition (per serving):

Calories: 50

Protein: 1g

Carbohydrates: 13g

Fat: 0g

Fiber: 0g

Sugar: 11g

3. Berry Coconut Electrolyte Drink

Ingredients:

- 1 cup mixed berries (strawberries, blueberries, raspberries)
- 2 cups coconut water
- 1/4 teaspoon sea salt
- 1 tablespoon honey or maple syrup
- 1 cup cold water

Directions:

1. In a blender, combine the mixed berries, coconut water, sea salt, and honey or maple syrup.
2. Blend until smooth.
3. Strain the mixture through a fine-mesh sieve into a pitcher to remove any pulp.
4. Add the cold water and stir well.
5. Chill in the refrigerator for at least 1 hour before serving.
6. Serve over ice if desired.

Serving Size:

4 servings

Nutrition (per serving):

Calories: 50

Protein: 1g

Carbohydrates: 13g

Fat: 0g

Fiber: 1g

Sugar: 11g

4. Pineapple Ginger Electrolyte Drink

Ingredients:

- 1 cup pineapple juice (fresh or no added sugar)
- 1/2 teaspoon grated fresh ginger
- 2 cups coconut water
- 1/4 teaspoon sea salt
- 1 tablespoon honey or agave syrup
- 1 cup cold water

Directions:

1. In a blender, combine the pineapple juice, grated ginger, coconut water, sea salt, and honey or agave syrup.
2. Blend until smooth.
3. Strain the mixture through a fine-mesh sieve into a pitcher to remove any pulp or ginger fibers.
4. Add the cold water and stir well.
5. Chill in the refrigerator for at least 1 hour before serving.
6. Serve over ice if desired.

Serving Size:

4 servings

Nutrition (per serving):

Calories: 60

Protein: 0g

Carbohydrates: 15g

Fat: 0g

Fiber: 0g

Sugar: 14g

5. Green Apple Electrolyte Drink

Ingredients:

- 2 green apples (juiced or blended and strained)
- 2 cups coconut water
- 1/4 teaspoon sea salt
- 1 tablespoon honey or agave syrup
- 1 cup cold water
- Juice of 1 lemon

Directions:

1. Juice the green apples or blend them and strain the juice into a pitcher.
2. Add the coconut water, sea salt, honey or agave syrup, and lemon juice.
3. Stir well until everything is fully dissolved and combined.
4. Add the cold water and stir again.
5. Chill in the refrigerator for at least 1 hour before serving.
6. Serve over ice if desired.

Serving Size:

4 servings

Nutrition (per serving):

Calories: 60

Protein: 0g

Carbohydratcs: 15g

Fat: 0g

Fiber: 0g
Sugar: 13g

8.2 Herbal Teas for Relaxation

1. Chamomile Lavender Tea

Ingredients:

- 2 teaspoons dried chamomile flowers
- 1 teaspoon dried lavender buds
- 2 cups boiling water
- Honey or lemon (optional, for taste)

Directions:

1. Place the dried chamomile flowers and lavender buds in a teapot or infuser.
2. Pour the boiling water over the herbs.
3. Let steep for 5-10 minutes.
4. Strain the tea into cups.
5. Add honey or lemon if desired.
6. Serve warm.

Serving Size:

2 servings

Nutrition (per serving):

Calories: 2

Protein: 0g

Carbohydrates: 0g

Fat: 0g

Fiber: 0g

Sugar: 0g

2. Peppermint Valerian Root Tea

Ingredients:

- 2 teaspoons dried peppermint leaves
- 1 teaspoon dried valerian root
- 2 cups boiling water
- Honey (optional, for taste)

Directions:

1. Place the dried peppermint leaves and valerian root in a teapot or infuser.
2. Pour the boiling water over the herbs.
3. Let steep for 5-7 minutes.
4. Strain the tea into cups.
5. Add honey if desired.
6. Serve warm.

Serving Size:

2 servings

Nutrition (per serving):

Calories: 2

Protein: 0g

Carbohydrates: 0g

Fat: 0g

Fiber: 0g

Sugar: 0g

3. Lemon Balm and Passionflower Tea

Ingredients:

- 2 teaspoons dried lemon balm leaves
- 1 teaspoon dried passionflower
- 2 cups boiling water
- Lemon slice or honey (optional, for taste)

Directions:

1. Place the dried lemon balm leaves and passionflower in a teapot or infuser.
2. Pour the boiling water over the herbs.
3. Let steep for 5-10 minutes.
4. Strain the tea into cups.
5. Add a lemon slice or honey if desired.
6. Serve warm.

Serving Size:

2 servings

Nutrition (per serving):

Calories: 2

Protein: 0g

Carbohydrates: 0g

Fat: 0g

Fiber: 0g

Sugar: 0g

4. Holy Basil (Tulsi) Tea

Ingredients:

- 2 teaspoons dried holy basil (Tulsi) leaves
- 2 cups boiling water
- Honey or lemon (optional, for taste)

Directions:

1. Place the dried holy basil leaves in a teapot or infuser.
2. Pour the boiling water over the leaves.
3. Let steep for 5-10 minutes.
4. Strain the tea into cups.
5. Add honey or lemon if desired.
6. Serve warm.

Serving Size:

2 servings

Nutrition (per serving):

Calories: 2

Protein: 0g

Carbohydrates: 0g

Fat: 0g

Fiber: 0g

Sugar: 0g

5. Rooibos and Vanilla Tea

Ingredients:

- 2 teaspoons rooibos tea leaves

- 1 vanilla bean (split) or 1 teaspoon vanilla extract
- 2 cups boiling water
- Honey (optional, for taste)

Directions:

1. Place the rooibos tea leaves and the split vanilla bean (or vanilla extract) in a teapot or infuser.
2. Pour the boiling water over the tea leaves and vanilla.
3. Let steep for 5-7 minutes.
4. Strain the tea into cups.
5. Add honey if desired.
6. Serve warm.

Serving Size:

2 servings

Nutrition (per serving):

Calories: 2
Protein: 0g
Carbohydrates: 0g
Fat: 0g
Fiber: 0g
Sugar: 0g

8.3 Smoothies for Sustained Energy

1. Green Power Smoothie

Ingredients:

- 1 cup spinach
- 1 banana
- 1/2 avocado
- 1 cup unsweetened almond milk
- 1 tablespoon chia seeds
- 1 tablespoon honey or maple syrup
- 1/2 cup ice

Directions:

1. Add all ingredients to a blender.
2. Blend until smooth.
3. Serve immediately.

Serving Size:

1 serving

Nutrition (per serving):

Calories: 300

Protein: 4g

Carbohydrates: 47g

Fat: 12g

Fiber: 10g

Sugar: 20g

2. Berry Banana Smoothie

Ingredients:

- 1 cup mixed berries (strawberries, blueberries, raspberries)
- 1 banana
- 1 cup Greek yogurt
- 1/2 cup orange juice
- 1 tablespoon flaxseeds
- 1/2 cup ice

Directions:

1. Add all ingredients to a blender.
2. Blend until smooth.
3. Serve immediately.

Serving Size:

1 serving

Nutrition (per serving):

Calories: 280

Protein: 10g

Carbohydrates: 52g

Fat: 5g

Fiber: 9g

Sugar: 32g

3. Peanut Butter Banana Smoothie

Ingredients:

- 1 banana

- 2 tablespoons peanut butter
- 1 cup unsweetened almond milk
- 1 tablespoon honey or maple syrup
- 1 scoop vanilla protein powder
- 1/2 cup ice

Directions:

1. Add all ingredients to a blender.
2. Blend until smooth.
3. Serve immediately.
4. Serving Size:

1 serving

Nutrition (per serving):

Calories: 400
Protein: 25g
Carbohydrates: 40g
Fat: 18g
Fiber: 5g
Sugar: 22g

4. Tropical Energy Smoothie

Ingredients:

- 1 cup pineapple chunks
- 1/2 mango (peeled and diced)
- 1 banana
- 1 cup coconut water
- 1 tablespoon hemp seeds

- 1/2 cup ice

Directions:

1. Add all ingredients to a blender.
2. Blend until smooth.
3. Serve immediately.

Serving Size:

1 serving

Nutrition (per serving):

Calories: 260
Protein: 4g
Carbohydrates: 63g
Fat: 2g
Fiber: 7g
Sugar: 45g

5. Chocolate Almond Smoothie

Ingredients:

- 1 banana
- 1 tablespoon almond butter
- 1 cup unsweetened almond milk
- 1 tablespoon cocoa powder
- 1 scoop chocolate protein powder
- 1/2 cup ice

Directions:

1. Add all ingredients to a blender.

2. Blend until smooth.

3. Serve immediately.

Serving Size:

1 serving

Nutrition (per serving):

Calories: 350

Protein: 25g

Carbohydrates: 40g

Fat: 12g

Fiber: 7g

Sugar: 20g

8.4 Homemade Infused Waters

1. Lemon Mint Infused Water

Ingredients:

- 1 lemon, thinly sliced
- 10 fresh mint leaves
- 1 liter (4 cups) cold water
- Ice cubes (optional)

Directions:

1. Place the lemon slices and mint leaves in a large pitcher.
2. Pour the cold water over the lemon and mint.
3. Stir gently to combine.
4. Refrigerate for at least 2 hours to allow the flavors to infuse.
5. Serve chilled, with ice cubes if desired.

Serving Size:

4 servings (1 cup each)

Nutrition (per serving):

Calories: 2

Protein: 0g

Carbohydrates: 1g

Fat: 0g

Fiber: 0g

Sugar: 0g

2. Cucumber Basil Infused Water

Ingredients:

- 1/2 cucumber, thinly sliced
- 10 fresh basil leaves
- 1 liter (4 cups) cold water
- Ice cubes (optional)

Directions:

1. Place the cucumber slices and basil leaves in a large pitcher.
2. Pour the cold water over the cucumber and basil.
3. Stir gently to combine.
4. Refrigerate for at least 2 hours to allow the flavors to infuse.
5. Serve chilled, with ice cubes if desired.

Serving Size:

4 servings (1 cup each)

Nutrition (per serving):

Calories: 1

Protein: 0g

Carbohydrates: 0g

Fat: 0g

Fiber: 0g

Sugar: 0g

3. Strawberry Lime Infused Water

Ingredients:

- 1/2 cup strawberries, hulled and sliced

- 1 lime, thinly sliced
- 1 liter (4 cups) cold water
- Ice cubes (optional)

Directions:

1. Place the strawberry slices and lime slices in a large pitcher.
2. Pour the cold water over the strawberries and lime.
3. Stir gently to combine.
4. Refrigerate for at least 2 hours to allow the flavors to infuse.
5. Serve chilled, with ice cubes if desired.

Serving Size:

4 servings (1 cup each)

Nutrition (per serving):

Calories: 3
Protein: 0g
Carbohydrates: 1g
Fat: 0g
Fiber: 0g
Sugar: 0g

4. Orange Ginger Infused Water

Ingredients:

- 1 orange, thinly sliced
- 1-inch piece of fresh ginger, thinly sliced
- 1 liter (4 cups) cold water
- Ice cubes (optional)

Directions:

1. Place the orange slices and ginger slices in a large pitcher.
2. Pour the cold water over the orange and ginger.
3. Stir gently to combine.
4. Refrigerate for at least 2 hours to allow the flavors to infuse.
5. Serve chilled, with ice cubes if desired.

Serving Size:

4 servings (1 cup each)

Nutrition (per serving):

Calories: 5

Protein: 0g

Carbohydrates: 1g

Fat: 0g

Fiber: 0g

Sugar: 1g

5. Blueberry Lavender Infused Water

Ingredients:

- 1/2 cup blueberries
- 1 teaspoon dried lavender buds
- 1 liter (4 cups) cold water
- Ice cubes (optional)

Directions:

1. Place the blueberries and dried lavender buds in a large pitcher.
2. Pour the cold water over the blueberries and lavender.

3. Stir gently to combine.

4. Refrigerate for at least 2 hours to allow the flavors to infuse.

5. Serve chilled, with ice cubes if desired.

Serving Size:

4 servings (1 cup each)

Nutrition (per serving):

Calories: 2

Protein: 0g

Carbohydrates: 1g

Fat: 0g

Fiber: 0g

Sugar: 0g

Chapter 9: Meal Plans and Shopping Lists

9.1 7-Day POTS-Friendly Meal Plan

Day 1

Breakfast: Green Power Smoothie

Lunch: Hearty Salad with Electrolyte-Rich Ingredients

Snack: Electrolyte-Boosting Snack

Dinner: Balanced One-Pot Meal

Dessert: Low-Sugar Treat

Day 2

Breakfast: Berry Banana Smoothie

Lunch: Light and Easy Sandwich

Snack: High-Fiber Snack Bar

Dinner: Lean Protein Entree

Dessert: Hydrating Gelatin Dessert

Day 3

Breakfast: Peanut Butter Banana Smoothie

Lunch: Protein-Packed Wrap

Snack: Hydrating Fruit and Veggie Snack

Dinner: Flavorful and Hydrating Stew

Dessert: Protein-Rich Pudding

Day 4

Breakfast: Tropical Energy Smoothie

Lunch: Hearty Salad with Electrolyte-Rich Ingredients

Snack: Easy-to-Make Smoothie Bowl

Dinner: Balanced One-Pot Meal

Dessert: Fresh and Fruity Dessert

Day 5
Breakfast: Chocolate Almond Smoothie
Lunch: Warm and Comforting Soup
Snack: Electrolyte-Rich Drink
Dinner: Lean Protein Entree
Dessert: Low-Sugar Treat

Day 6
Breakfast: Balanced Breakfast Bowl
Lunch: Protein-Packed Wrap
Snack: High-Fiber Snack Bar
Dinner: Flavorful and Hydrating Stew
Dessert: Hydrating Gelatin Dessert

Day 7
Breakfast: Green Power Smoothie
Lunch: Light and Easy Sandwich
Snack: Hydrating Fruit and Veggie Snack
Dinner: Balanced One-Pot Meal
Dessert: Fresh and Fruity Dessert

9.2 Grocery Shopping Tips

1. Plan Your Meals:

Before heading to the store, create a weekly meal plan. This helps you stay organized and ensures you have all necessary ingredients for your POTS-friendly meals.
2. Make a Detailed Shopping List:

Write down all ingredients needed for your meal plan. Categorize items by sections of the store (produce, dairy, grains, etc.) to streamline your shopping trip.
3. Focus on Hydration:

Incorporate hydrating food varieties like cucumbers, watermelon, oranges, and strawberries. These foods help maintain hydration levels throughout the day.
4. Choose Electrolyte-Rich Foods:

Opt for foods high in electrolytes, such as bananas, avocados, spinach, and coconut water. These can help manage blood pressure and hydration.
5. Opt for Whole Foods:

Select whole, unprocessed foods. Fresh fruits, vegetables, lean proteins, whole grains, nuts, and seeds should be the bulk of your groceries.
6. Prioritize Lean Proteins:

Incorporate sources like chicken, turkey, fish, beans, lentils, and tofu. These proteins help maintain energy and muscle mass.
7. Include Healthy Fats:

Add avocados, nuts, seeds, and olive oil to your list. These fats are beneficial for overall health and can help with satiety.

8. Avoid High-Sodium and Processed Foods:

Check labels and steer clear of foods with high sodium content and added preservatives, as these can worsen POTS symptoms.
9. Stock Up on High-Fiber Foods:

Choose whole grains, vegetables, fruits, and legumes. High-fiber foods aid in digestion and help maintain stable blood sugar levels.
10. Look for Convenient Options:

Pre-cut vegetables, ready-to-eat salads, and pre-cooked grains can save time and energy, making it easier to prepare nutritious meals.

Chapter 10: Supplements and Hydration

10.1 Essential Supplements for POTS

While a balanced diet is crucial for managing POTS (Postural Orthostatic Tachycardia Syndrome), certain supplements can help fill nutritional gaps and support overall health. Here are some essential supplements for POTS patients:

1. Electrolyte Supplements:

Electrolytes such as sodium, potassium, magnesium, and calcium are vital for maintaining fluid balance and proper nerve and muscle function. Enhancements can help in the event that dietary admission is lacking.
2. Vitamin B12:

Vitamin B12 supports nerve health and energy production. POTS patients, especially those with absorption issues, may benefit from B12 supplements.
3. Omega-3 Fatty Acids:

Omega-3s, found in fish oil supplements, have anti-inflammatory properties and support heart and brain health.
4. Vitamin D:

Vitamin D is important for bone health and immune function. Many people are deficient, and supplementation can be beneficial, especially if sunlight exposure is limited.

5. Coenzyme Q10 (CoQ10):

CoQ10 is involved in energy production at the cellular level and may help reduce fatigue and improve exercise tolerance in POTS patients.

6. L-Carnitine:

L-Carnitine helps transport fatty acids into the mitochondria for energy production and may help improve symptoms of fatigue.

7. Iron:

Iron is essential for oxygen transport in the blood. POTS patients with anemia or low iron levels might need supplements to boost their iron stores.

Always consult with a healthcare provider before starting any new supplements to ensure they are appropriate for your individual health needs and conditions.

10.2 Hydration Strategies

Proper hydration is crucial for managing POTS (Postural Orthostatic Tachycardia Syndrome) as it helps maintain blood volume and pressure, reducing symptoms like dizziness and fatigue. Here are some effective hydration strategies:

1. Drink Plenty of Fluids:

Plan to polish off something like 2-3 liters of water everyday. Spread out your fluid intake throughout the day to maintain consistent hydration levels.
2. Incorporate Electrolyte-Rich Drinks:

Include beverages like coconut water, sports drinks, or homemade electrolyte solutions. These drinks help replenish electrolytes lost through sweat and urine, maintaining proper fluid balance.
3. Eat Hydrating Foods:

Polish off products of the soil with high water content, like cucumbers, watermelon, oranges, and strawberries. These foods contribute to overall hydration and provide essential nutrients.
4. Use Salt:

Increasing salt intake can help retain fluids and maintain blood volume. Use a salt shaker liberally on your food or consider salt tablets if recommended by your healthcare provider.
5. Avoid Dehydrating Substances:

Limit consumption of caffeine and alcohol as they can increase urine output and contribute to dehydration.

6. Carry a Water Bottle:

Keep a water bottle with you at all times to remind yourself to drink regularly. Sipping water consistently can help maintain steady hydration levels.

7. Monitor Urine Color:

Use pee tone as a basic mark of hydration status. Pale yellow urine typically indicates good hydration, while darker urine suggests a need for more fluids.

By following these strategies, you can help manage POTS symptoms and support overall well-being through effective hydration.

Chapter 11: Lifestyle Tips for Managing POTS

11.1 Exercise and Physical Activity

Exercise and physical activity play a crucial role in managing POTS (Postural Orthostatic Tachycardia Syndrome) by improving cardiovascular fitness, increasing blood flow to the brain and muscles, and enhancing overall well-being. Here are a few central issues to consider:

1. Start Gradually:

Begin with low-impact exercises such as walking, swimming, or stationary cycling. Progressively increment force and length as endured.
2. Focus on Cardiovascular Fitness:

Aerobic exercises like jogging, dancing, or rowing can improve heart and lung function, helping to reduce symptoms of dizziness and fatigue.
3. Incorporate Strength Training:

Include resistance exercises using body weight, resistance bands, or light weights to strengthen muscles. Strong muscles can assist in maintaining posture and reducing joint pain.
4. Monitor Symptoms:

Focus on how your body answers work out. Track symptoms like dizziness, fatigue, or palpitations. Adjust intensity or duration as needed to avoid exacerbating symptoms.

5. Stay Consistent:

Aim for regular exercise sessions throughout the week. Consistency is key to improving cardiovascular fitness and reaping long-term benefits.

6. Use Postural Techniques:

Incorporate techniques like compression garments or gradual changes in posture to minimize orthostatic intolerance during and after exercise.

7. Work with a Physical Therapist:

A physical therapist can create a tailored exercise program and provide guidance on proper techniques and progression based on your individual needs and capabilities.

8. Stay Hydrated:

Drink plenty of fluids before, during, and after exercise to maintain hydration and support cardiovascular function.

9. Listen to Your Body:

Respect your body's limits and rest when needed. Avoid overexertion, especially during periods of symptom exacerbation or flare-ups.

By incorporating regular exercise and physical activity into your routine, you can enhance your overall health, manage POTS symptoms more effectively, and improve your quality of life. Always consult with your healthcare provider before starting a new exercise program, especially if you have underlying health conditions or concerns.

11.2 Stress Management Techniques

Managing stress is important for individuals with POTS (Postural Orthostatic Tachycardia Syndrome) as stress can exacerbate symptoms such as increased heart rate and blood pressure fluctuations. Here are some straightforward pressure the board procedures:

1. Deep Breathing Exercises:

Practice profound breathing procedures to advance unwinding and lessen nervousness. Center around sluggish, full breaths, breathing in through your nose and breathing out through your mouth.
2. Meditation and Mindfulness:

Integrate contemplation or care rehearses into your everyday daily practice. These techniques help calm the mind and improve stress resilience.
3. Gentle Exercise:

Engage in gentle exercises like yoga or tai chi, which combine physical movement with mindfulness and relaxation techniques.
4. Progressive Muscle Relaxation:

Tense and afterward loosen up each muscle bunch in your body, beginning from your toes up to your head. This method helps discharge actual strain and advance unwinding.
5. Maintain a Healthy Lifestyle:

Prioritize adequate sleep, a balanced diet, and regular physical activity to support overall well-being and reduce stress levels.
6. Seek Social Support:

Stay connected with friends, family, or support groups. Sharing experiences and receiving emotional support can help alleviate stress.

7. Practice Time Management:

Organize tasks and prioritize activities to minimize feelings of overwhelm. Break tasks into smaller, manageable steps to reduce stress associated with deadlines or responsibilities.
8. Limit Stimulants:

Reduce consumption of caffeine and alcohol, as these can increase feelings of anxiety and worsen POTS symptoms.

Incorporating these stress management techniques into your daily routine can help you better cope with stress, reduce symptom severity, and improve overall quality of life with POTS.

Chapter 12: Staying Motivated and Connected

12.1 Maintaining Long-Term Dietary Changes

Maintaining long-term dietary changes is essential for managing POTS (Postural Orthostatic Tachycardia Syndrome) effectively and improving overall health. Here are a few hints to assist you with supporting good dieting propensities:

1. Establish Realistic Goals:

Put forth attainable objectives that line up with your wellbeing needs and way of life. Begin with little changes and continuously integrate new propensities over the long run.
2. Focus on Balanced Nutrition:

Stress a reasonable eating routine wealthy in organic products, vegetables, lean proteins, entire grains, and solid fats. This ensures you receive essential nutrients to support overall well-being.
3. Plan Ahead:

Plan your feasts and snacks ahead of time to stay away from rash food decisions. Use grocery lists and meal prepping to simplify healthy eating throughout the week.
4. Find Healthy Substitutions:

Identify healthier alternatives to your favorite foods. For example, swap refined grains for whole grains, or opt for baked instead of fried options.
5. Practice Mindful Eating:

Focus on craving and totality signs, and appreciate each chomp. Eating mindfully can help prevent overeating and promote better digestion.

6. Stay Hydrated:

Drink an adequate amount of water throughout the day to maintain hydration levels and support overall health.

7. Seek Professional Guidance:

Consult with a registered dietitian or healthcare provider for personalized dietary advice and support. They can help you navigate dietary challenges and make sustainable choices.

8. Stay Consistent:

Consistency is key to maintaining long-term dietary changes. Focus on making healthy eating a habit rather than a short-term fix.

9. Celebrate Progress:

Acknowledge and celebrate your achievements along the way. Reward yourself for sticking to your dietary goals and milestones.

By incorporating these strategies into your daily routine, you can establish and maintain long-term dietary changes that support your health and well-being with POTS.